A YEAR WITHOUT FOOD

DISCOVER THE UNIMAGINABLE WORLD OF PROVEN ENERGETIC NOURISHMENT

RAY MAOR

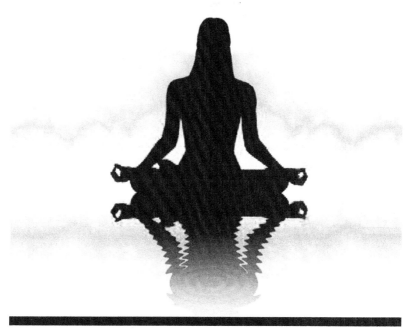

A YEAR WITHOUT FOOD

Published by
Aingeal Rose and Ahonu
Twin Flame Productions LLC

DISCOVER THE UNIMAGINABLE WORLD
OF PROVEN ENERGETIC NOURISHMENT

A Year Without Food
Maor, Ray, 1981 –
A Year Without Food
Ray Maor.
ISBN-10: 1-880765-98-5
ISBN-13: 978-1-880765-98-2

Designed and Edited by: Aingeal Rose & Ahonu
https://aingealroseandahonu.com
Published by World of Empowerment Press,
an imprint of Twin Flame Productions LLC
https://twinflameproductions.us

Disclaimer

Ray Maor does not guarantee that solutions suggested in these materials will be effective in your particular situation. If you are not familiar with any of the steps listed in any solution, Ray Maor advises that you do not proceed without first consulting additional resources.

To the maximum extent permitted by applicable law, in no event shall Ray Maor, or his suppliers (or their respective agents, directors, employees or representatives) be liable for any damages whatsoever (including, without limitation, consequential, incidental, direct, indirect, special, economic, punitive or similar damages, or damages for loss of business profits, loss of goodwill, business interruption, computer failure or malfunction, loss of business information or any and all other commercial or pecuniary damages or losses) arising out of or in connection with the use of or inability to use the materials, including without limitation the use or performance of software or documents, the provision of or failure to provide services, or information available from this book or his websites, however caused and on any legal theory of liability (whether in tort, contract or otherwise), even if Ray Maor has been advised of the possibility of such damages or for any claim by any other party. Because some jurisdictions prohibit the exclusion or limitation of liability for consequential or incidental damages, the above limitation may not apply to you. Always consult a licensed health practitioner for all health issues. Full Terms & Conditions and Disclaimer at https://raymaor.com

Address all inquiries to:
Ray Maor,
Ezer Veitsman 10, Hod Hasharon, Israel

Table of Contents

RAY MAOR

After years of spiritual development in search of a higher understanding of his path, Ray Maor decided to take the ultimate consciousness leap and pass through a breatharian initiation process which completely transformed his life.

As a breatharian, he seeks to share this deep experience to promote human understanding of the spiritual/mental connection we have with our physical bodies and our capacity to surpass standard abilities.

Ray volunteered to be tested in a televised medical experiment for an investigative reporting show in July 2013. In the show, Ray subjected himself to going without food and water for eight days and was medically tested on a daily basis to prove that, as a breatharian, his blood composition would not change and his physical state would not be altered.

In this book, Ray Maor gives us his personal story and shares the information he has researched and collected about the energy of prana, the multiple benefits of a breatharian lifestyle and some life changing tips.

RAY MAOR

It is both an honor and privilege to publish this book about my breatharian journey—a journey that more and more people are undertaking every day. Since the beginning of my own breatharian initiation, I have had an inkling that my journey would lead me to shed light on subjects that are rarely discussed around a typical Saturday dinner table.

I have found only a few books that contain serious discussions about the breatharian lifestyle and initiation process. There may be others, but I have been disappointed by the general lack of information to satisfy the more scientific and logical thinkers among us.

To open a conversation with skeptics, I set out to prove what is possible. Following my exposure and after the long adaptation period to the lifestyle, it has been my goal to share my knowledge as a breatharian and offer some answers to the many questions elicited by the experiment. By writing this book, I hope to achieve this goal.

Ray Maor
Israel, October 2018

RAY MAOR

Ever since I can remember I have been a thrill seeker. As a child living in the desert of South Israel, I had a lot of time to ponder the meaning of life, who we are as people, *what* we are and what our purpose is in living in this world. Throughout my adolescence I achieved high scores in mathematics, physics and other sciences. At the age of eighteen I was mandatorily drafted into a special IT unit in the IDF (Israel Defense Forces) and subsequently signed a contract to remain in the IDF for a period of five full years (two additional years beyond the mandatory service). During this time, I became an officer in my unit and graduated with the rank of a lieutenant.

Coming to the end of my term of service, I realized that I was and still am a pacifist, and a great call for self-fulfillment arose in my heart. I set out on a quest to understand everything there is to understand about life and its deeper meanings. At the age of twenty-four, I travelled through South America for nine months and returned to Israel to work as a consultant in the IT world. At twenty-nine, I decided to travel for another year—this time a trip around the world and an experience that well and truly changed me by opening my mind and inspiring me to go in a completely new direction in life.

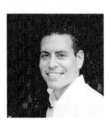

Fig. 1- Ray Maor

How This Book Came To Be

Many years ago, I heard of people known as *sungazers* who gaze at the sun to free themselves from their dependency on food. In those days I was skeptical, leaning towards a very left-brain perspective. I knew the sun to be a great source of energy, but did not believe human beings had the right equipment to be nourished by it in the way plants and trees are replenished through photosynthesis. It was not logical or even imaginable to me at that point in my life. I had to see things to believe them. Lacking evidence, I regarded sungazing and other superhuman phenomena to be misguided Internet rumors and quickly gave up my investigations into these groups.

Everything changed when I came back to Israel after my year-long trip around the world. I became involved with a community of spiritual activists formally known as *The Love Revolution*, which opened my mind and my heart. I was introduced to many interesting spiritual people as well as new concepts and belief systems. Among them was a special man named Tal. Since meeting Tal, he has become my dear friend and brother. As our relationship developed into friendship, he began to share with me the truths of his pranic lifestyle. Needless to say, what he told me blew my mind!

Here was Tal—living, breathing proof of pranic living in action that I could not ignore. My curiosity was piqued. I wanted to know more and so began my quest to fully understand this rare human ability.

A pranic/breatharian lifestyle is a lifestyle of independence from the daily necessity of food; a lifestyle in which we do not experience hunger or thirst, we have more energy, have a deeper connection to our inner guidance, to nature and to ourselves. Of course, I could not completely understand what it really meant to be a breatharian at the time. I still had many questions that needed to be answered.

However, the seed of interest had been planted and I knew right then that I would become a test subject and pioneer for this alternative way of being. It was as if my future self was calling me and saying, "Ray, you have already completed this process with success. This is your path and it will bring you great understanding."

Having Tal as a friend and advisor gave me an insider's perspective into this lifestyle. We spent a lot of time together at parties and festivals and I soon had to accept the truth: breatharian living is possible! It was especially important to me to see that it could be a functional lifestyle in the western world. To be a breatharian, one does not necessarily have to be a recluse, live like a hermit or be as holy as an Indian yogi. Today, our little breatharian circle of friends has expanded to include practitioners from all walks of life. My closest breatharian friends live in Tel-Aviv.

My point in presenting our 'normality' is for you to understand that this is not some miraculous and exclusive way of living. You can do anything if you focus and put your mind to it. One thing you, Tal and I have in common is that we each have a burning desire to maximize our potential. This is what drives us to read books on self-realization and to practice meditation. Outside of this we work, travel, have relationships and simply enjoy the pleasures of life. We are not monks who have renounced all earthly possessions or reclusive Indian yogis who meditate 24/7 on a Himalayan peak.

In this book, I tell my story and the preparations and processes I underwent to transition to a breatharian and my life as a guide with real-life examples of this lifestyle.

I know that you seekers will enjoy this book, otherwise it would not have found its way into your hands! Just remember one thing—this is *my* story. Each story has many variables and requires a hierarchy of conscious understanding. What I mean by this is that everything may not make sense right away; in fact, some things may seem quite illogical at first and conflict with your current set of beliefs. That is completely all right and I leave it up to you to decide which parts of the information *feel* right for you. All the answers you seek are already inside you and the only two words you should practice to completely integrate this information with your higher mind are *surrender* and *allow*. Surrender control to your higher, smarter self who knows who you are better than you know yourself and allow that part of yourself to lead you as it has done so many times without resistance from your small egoic fears.

Summary

In **Chapters One, Two and Three** I discuss the life force of *prana*, also known as *chi*, our ability to use it and how to raise it in our body via conscious belief systems. I speak about people who choose breatharian lifestyles and what defines them, as well as why this knowledge is not known to all.

In **Chapter Four** I explain why breatharians choose this lifestyle and concentrate on the spiritual and health benefits which come with it. I discuss different aspects of being a breatharian and the advantages I have seen manifest in my friends over the years.

In **Chapter Five** I discuss my personal story of discovery, choice and initiation. I detail my challenges and my inner call to make this knowledge available to the public.

In **Chapter Six** I delve into my television debut; the experience in which I volunteered to live for eight days without food or water under video surveillance, being medically monitored on a daily basis. Through this media exposure I became well-known which allowed me to connect with many curious souls who seek knowledge in the spiritual realms. (The show can be viewed on my website www.raymaor.com)

In **Chapter Seven** I explain the most commonly known methods of becoming a breatharian, including the method that I developed called *The Pranic Living Group Initiation*.

In **Chapter Eight** I discuss the mind-mastery that can be used to actively further one's personal development. I share a collection of tips and tricks that assist in understanding the way our minds work, how to control and influence them, how to reprogram them and how to become more consciously aware of oneself.

In **Chapters Nine through Fourteen** I discuss the different challenges of being a breatharian from my own point of view and through the collective experiences of other breatharians whom I have initiated. I also give theories, scientific facts and additional thoughts about the different subjects discussed throughout the book.

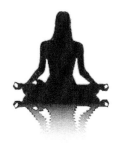

PART ONE

CHAPTER ONE

Prana

What Is Prana?

Prana is the energy that animates and connects all living beings. You may know this energy by other names such as: life force, liquid light, chi, the force, orgone and cosmic particles. The essence we try to convey with all these words is *universal life energy*. It is important to understand that with each inhalation, we are taking two things into our body—air and prana. Prana is the energy that drives all of life and is essential to our existence, more so than air.

In yoga, oriental medicine and martial arts, the term *prana* refers to cosmic energy believed to come from the sun and which connects all the elements in the universe. As the universal principle of energy or force responsible for the body's life, heat and maintenance, prana is the sum total of all the energy manifested in the universe. This life energy has been vividly invoked and described in the Vedas and in Ayurveda, Tantra and Tibetan medicine.

Prana is not only found in air; it exists everywhere. It is within me and you, in plants and animals, in the earth and all the elements that create our planet. There is no place where prana does not exist. It exists even in the spaces we perceive to be void. Pranic energy is closely connected to the energy one might describe as the *soul* and life cannot exist without it. There is an old saying that a man can live for forty days without food, three days without water, five minutes without oxygen but without prana, not even one second!

Prana is invisible to the human eye and not measurable with our current scientific instruments. Despite this, as spiritual individuals we can feel the truth of its existence all around us.

Prana moves through the body via an energy tube about the size of the circle between your index finger and thumb. This tube begins approximately ten centimeters above your head or crown chakra and continues downward through all seven chakras[1], finishing under the perineum located between the anus and the genitals. Prana is a subtle element pervading each cell in the living tissue and fluid of every organism, much like electricity through atoms in a battery.

Each person naturally maintains a different level of prana which varies from day to day. Generally, when you are in a place where you feel comfortable and in 'the present moment', you find you are not motivated to eat from habit or emotional need. For example, when you are happy, content or in love, you may notice your appetite tends to decrease. This is because in higher vibrational states of being, the percentage of prana in your body rises. In contrast, lower vibrational states such as melancholy, frustration, fear and dissatisfaction can cause you to eat much more than is absolutely necessary. As our percentage of prana decreases, we seek comfort in the pleasures of taste and texture.

Our prana percentage also depends on our environment. With air pollution increasing in many big cities, the percentage of prana in the air continues to decrease. Nature, on the other hand provides abundant prana, which is why you may also find yourself eating less in natural settings.

―――――――――――

[1] Chakras are invisible wheels of energy located at varying points along the spinal column in the energetic body of man. These wheels of energy break down sunlight and distribute specific colors to different organs for nourishment. The chakras are also portals to other dimensions and connect to our DNA strands. When the chakras are working in harmony with each other, they activate higher DNA strands and lead us to experiences of higher consciousness.

Prana is often discussed in martial art philosophies and many claim it provides conscious individuals with superhuman abilities. In India, yogis are known to practice Pranayama; specific sets of breathing exercises designed to draw additional prana into the body with each breath. Raising your personal level of prana is not very difficult and can be achieved through the regular practice of meditation, deep breathing exercises and conscious intention.

Prana is an important general discovery as we try to piece together the missing links in our human evolution. Because our current scientific instruments cannot measure prana, its existence is largely ignored or misunderstood. This is one of the reasons I decided to write this book after my years of personal research on the subject.

For more information on prana and the breatharian way of life, I have given a list of external resources at the end of the book.

CHAPTER TWO

The Scale Of Human Nutrition

The Scale Of Human Nutrition

Many different groups of people distinguish themselves from others by their dietary choices. Some pick their diets consciously, others not so much. Some diets are based on philosophy and religion while others are maintained purely for health and other physical reasons. To help put things in perspective, I have pieced together a scale of human nutrition.

Let's start with the *omnivore* whose diet today's society deems normal. An omnivore consumes both plant and animal materials, often without any specific eating philosophy. Sometimes omnivores refine their diets to control physical appearance or health, to build muscle, lose weight or lower cholesterol.

Next is the well-known *vegetarian* who chooses not to eat meat. This is often a religious or philosophical choice, demonstrating compassion for animals subjected to harsh practices in the meat industry. In recent years, research such as The China Study[2] has proved that excessive consumption of meat—more than three meals a week—is not as healthy for the human body as was once thought. This has provided new motivation for people to become vegetarian.

---

[2] The China Study (1st Edition, Hardback), ISBN 978-1932100389, publication date December 11, 2004.

Taking this a step further is the *vegan* who chooses to consume neither animals nor products derived from them including honey, dairy and eggs. Then there is the *raw foodist* who eats mostly fruits, nuts and vegetables in their natural raw form. This food philosophy encourages the consumption of food not heated above 40 °C because cooking heat damages the delicate nutrients and enzymes which nourish the body and aid digestion. Some raw foodists choose to go even deeper into the mechanics of the digestion process by following the rules of proper food combinations.

Following the raw food movement are lesser-known practitioners such as *fruitarians* who choose to be nourished solely from unprocessed fruits and *liquidarians* who blend raw food into soups and smoothies. Of course, individuals follow each of these diets to varying degrees. Some vegetarians eat fish, some vegans consume honey and some raw foodists enjoy a cooked meal from time to time. Levels of commitment are entirely up to individuals.

In general, the further along a person is on this scale, the easier it is for their digestive system to function and the cleaner and healthier their body becomes. These lifestyles also free up energy to perform other activities. Today most diseases are caused by bad nutrition and body toxicity. Until about 150 years ago, the human race only consumed fresh food. More recent inventions like pesticides, chemical preservatives, high sugar concentrates, chemical sugar replacements, fast food and the increase in food processing has thrown our alkaline/acid dietary balances way out of proportion. In a nutshell, our body needs an 80:20 (or at least 60:40) balance of alkaline to acid compounds to thrive. For the most part, fruits and vegetables are alkaline while meat, bread and other wheat/grain products, dairy and sugary foods contribute to acidity and toxicity in the body.

Many spiritual seekers naturally feel called to climb higher along this scale of nutrition towards vegetarian/vegan/raw food/fruitarian/liquidarian ways of life.

While the initial motivation may be to accept responsibility for the mistreatment of animals, it soon develops into a deeper understanding. Our body is our temple and what we allow into the body has an impact on the mind-body-spirit connection. The more you take care of your body, the easier it is to progress along your spiritual path.

The above scale describes most of the human race; people who consume food to satisfy both hunger and nutritional needs. There is no judgment here, just a statement of the facts most people tend to take for granted. For most people, food equals survival; there is no choice and they feel the need to consume a certain amount of food daily. The daily intake of vitamins, minerals, proteins, carbohydrates and many other nutrients must be in balance to provide sustainable energy sources for the body. This makes sense, though the general consciousness is pushing more and more towards greater health. Over recent years, more people have been making vegetarian and vegan choices and it is important to recognize how this goes hand in hand with the growth of our collective consciousness towards a healthier path.

The two most common types of 'light eaters' are *breatharians* and *sungazers* (who focus on the rising and setting sun to collect pranic nourishment). Breatharians get nutrition from a source other than food and exist on a completely different scale; they do not need to consume physical food for nourishment. Instead, they live directly off the life force or prana. Some breatharians live 100% off prana and do not even need to drink water! I am aware of only two people who live this way.

Perhaps you have heard of breatharians who live in India or Brazil following very disciplined spiritual paths. Let it be known that there are also breatharians such as myself who live in urban cities and maintain regular, modern, day-to-day lifestyles.

In order to simplify the differences, I have created a short table that describes the main differences between the two lifestyles.

People who derive nourishment from food:	People who derive nourishment from prana:
feel the sensations of hunger and thirst which arise when the body requires energy	do not feel hunger or thirst from nutritional need, though sensations may arise when bothered by negative emotions
require a nutritious diet of balanced vitamins and minerals	do not require additional balance because prana automatically provides the body with the nutrients required for optimum functioning; they will eat/ drink mostly according to taste and flavor or because of social requirements
have a large variety of food and tastes to choose from and consume an average of 3 meals per day	drastically limit themselves according to personal rules of the game.
experience **weight changes** according to diet and health habits; most people carry excessive fat in their bodies because they treat the body to be like a convenience store: A regular store will have a supply room in the back of just the right size to hold just the right number of supplies. Having too large an amount of supplies or too big a supply room makes it hard to find individual items, and requires more hands to do the work of accumulating, gathering, and storing. The body needs a supply room that is neither too big nor too small, but perfect. If it is too big you need extra work to maintain it, if it is too small you may prematurely run out of stock (energy). Relating this to the human body means having just the right amount of additional supplies (fat), and nothing more.	experience **ideal weight** according to what is best for the body because pranic energy 'fills' whatever is missing: This will hold true if he/she does not start eating a lot again in which case the body will get re-accustomed to receiving its nutrients via food and will stop its pranic intake (at different levels)

There are many additional differences discussed throughout this book.

CHAPTER THREE

Who Or What Is A Breatharian?

What Is A Breatharian?

A breatharian is a person who chooses to live mostly or completely from pranic nourishment. A breatharian does not need food to survive. However, they will probably choose to continue 'tasting' food for pleasure. A breatharian has escaped the hunger-compensation cycle completely and is free from food dependency.

The two processes currently known to me that allow one to become a breatharian are sungazing and pranic nourishment via the pranic living process. These transformational processes are discussed in later chapters. Each of these processes naturally increases the percentage of prana in the body and if an individual persists, the intake can increase up to 100%. Most people have less than 10% prana in their bodies and they run on electricity and need to be plugged into food for energy. By contrast, a breatharian runs on wireless solar power.

Currently, there are approximately 50,000 people who have undergone the pranic living process. Unfortunately, due to the challenges which this lifestyle entails (see Chapter 11), many people do not persist in this choice. There are only a few thousand practicing breatharians in the world. Despite this, the pranic living process itself can be a very positive life-changing event even if you do not continue to follow a breatharian lifestyle. It is getting increasing attention as more and more people become seekers of knowledge, looking for ways to be healthier and experience life more fully.

Most choose to eat or drink in small quantities, but not regularly. This practice is not based on a *need* to eat, but a desire to experience taste and texture or to fulfill social commitments. I calculate that a breatharian consumes between zero and one-third of his/her original recommended caloric intake because they no longer need to balance the body with nutrients. The pranic living process itself changes and balances the four physical, mental, emotional and spiritual bodies. That being said, a sensation of hunger can be triggered by negative emotional states.

I proved to surprised doctors through my television exposure that contrary to current scientific belief, my blood composition did not change when I stopped eating and drinking. I neither felt weak nor was I bedridden. The breatharian way of life is thus an option open to whoever is willing to take on the challenge and receive its many advantages but it is generally not suitable, appetizing or lasting for the majority of people alive today (more about this in Chapter 6).

Why Is It Not Common Knowledge?

The breatharian population is made up of only a few thousand people scattered across the globe, therefore the social proof of their existence remains nearly mythological. Most people who do not personally know a breatharian have closed mindsets about the possibility of their innate existence. In other words, they refuse to believe what they cannot see for themselves. In my personal experience, when I tell someone new that I do not eat, we initially both laugh because it does not make much sense. Only after a few minutes when the person sees that I am sane, can I actually let him or her know that I am not joking. It is always interesting to see how the conversation continues from there.

An Uncommon Lifestyle

After the television exposure, it became much easier for me to explain this lifestyle to people. I also started eating two or three meals a week, which helped. To most people, I just say that the body can learn to live on very little. To those who seek a higher and more complete understanding, I explain it more thoroughly like I do in this book. The television exposure helped to turn the *Is it possible?* question into *How is it possible?*

Insufficient Scientific Research

Let's face it—science does not like to address things it cannot explain. Even when concrete scientific data on the breatharian way of life is produced, it is unlikely that it will make headlines. Why? Proof of the existence of breatharians would call for a complete overhaul of the way science perceives and explains the normative functions of the human body. Thousands of books would have to be rewritten to acknowledge the amazing abilities of human consciousness. For this reason alone, scientists and doctors generally prefer to put the subject aside as if it is a joke.

Science, let's not forget, is missing a lot of information. It is hard to ignore that there is a big missing link in our theory[3] of evolution and we still have not discovered the origin of the first self-cloning biological cell. In fact, we have no idea how life began. Science also cannot tell us if our thoughts are created in the brain.

That being said, studies have been conducted on the breatharian way of life. The most famous one concentrates on an elder Indian man called Prahad Jani. The other scientific study conducted on me is described in Chapter 6. You can also see it online at www.raymaor.com.

The Breatharian Character

Most breatharians do not seek an audience; they just want to be left alone to enjoy their lives. This is a key reason why the breatharian lifestyle is not better known. Furthermore, most breatharian personalities are naturally introverted, seeking comfort in nature and distance from society.

---

[3] It is only a theory because it has not been completely proven with actual facts. However, in our school and colleges it is taught as facts. I am not arguing that some of it is true, but digging deeper, we find that things are missing.

When one knows oneself as intimately as this process encourages, one becomes humble and there is no egoistic need to prove oneself to others. In addition, most people do not understand—and sometimes do not *want* to understand. They find the truth too confronting. Perhaps they will accept the possibility after spending several consecutive days with a breatharian, watching he or she live and breathe (or more accurately, not eat) with their own eyes.

However, even then their logical minds may still refuse to accept this as a real possibility and they will work hard to find alternative reasons as to why it is impossible. As a breatharian, you come to understand there are different levels of acceptance and understanding for different individuals.

This is precisely why I have decided to share my experiences and make the subject more public. I realize that I may be called a heretic or a liar. I also know that I am strong enough to deal with the initial ridicule the subject inevitably evokes in western society.

As a breatharian, it is my intention to demonstrate the fullness of our human potential and what is possible. We unfortunately live in a society that highly underestimates the individual capacity for greatness. The truth is, our body is a vessel for something much greater, stronger and awesome than society would have you believe. However, we cannot begin to understand this until we transcend the illusions that keep us living in survival mode and the limits imposed by society's low expectations of what it means to be human. Know this: *you are a soul, not a body* and with the power of your mind you can create your own reality.

CHAPTER FOUR

The Many Benefits of a
Breatharian Lifestyle

Benefits Of

Breatharianism

Becoming a breatharian presents a great and exciting challenge to the spiritual seeker. It is a lifestyle choice not to be lightly undertaken and should only be pursued by people who feel a genuine inner calling. If you can accept that a pranic lifestyle is possible and if you have the desire to connect to a higher calling to push yourself to your own maximum potential, you might be ready to become one. You should however, understand that such a journey requires you to appreciate a power greater than yourself—whether you call it God, Spirit, Higher Self or any other name that describes faith in a greater power.

It is also important to recognize that becoming a breatharian is not the same as committing to an endless fast. This is what many people fail to understand when they first hear about this lifestyle. Breatharians have simply traded the traditional nutritional source of food for a purer source called prana.

This may sound daunting and difficult but from my own experience, I can say it is much easier than you may think. Don't let your imagination and anxiety get the better of you!

Most people are afraid of fasting without ever having experienced it; simply the idea keeps them from entertaining a breatharian lifestyle. People who complete a fast often recount that it was much easier than they expected, *as long as they maintained the right mindset.*

Many breatharians undergo one of the known breatharian initiations (discussed in Chapter 7), like the Pranic Living Group Initiation, simply for the experience and then go back to eating normally soon after. Remember, this is not a one-way track and no one expects you to make a lifelong commitment. The process of transformation itself has enormous benefits for personal development, so if you are interested in undergoing the process even just once, I recommend that you continue your own research and find a guide or a group to assist you. The pranic initiation is easier than most people think. The real challenge starts right after, but this lifestyle brings many gifts and is totally worth it! I have categorized these gifts into four sections: Health Benefits, Individual Benefits, Spiritual Benefits and Environmental Benefits.

Health Benefits

Longevity—Enjoy A Longer, Better Life!

Caloric Restriction (CR)[4] studies show that mammals who decrease their food intake by one third to one half can expect a 20%-30% longer life span. They also experience reduced cardiovascular risks and improved memory function.

Benefits Derived From CR Diets

CR in Primates—An ongoing study on rhesus macaques funded by The National Institute on Aging was initiated in 1989 at the University of Wisconsin. The 2009 results showed that caloric restriction in rhesus monkeys slowed down aging and significantly delayed the onset of age-related disorders such as cancer, diabetes, cardiovascular disease and brain atrophy. Eighty percent of the calorie-restricted monkeys were still alive at the end of the experiment compared to only half of the controls[5].

---

[4] 2 Caloric restriction is a field in scientific research where the food intake of a biological entity is minimized by half to one third to check its impact on the organism. A group of people living in California has decided to follow this as a way of life. See the Wikipedia entry for calorie restriction for more information.

[5] Wade, Nicholas (10 July 2009). "Dieting Moneys Offer Hope for Living Longer". New York Times. Retrieved 2009-09-10.

Lifespan

Seventy years ago C M McCay et al. discovered that reducing the number of calories fed to rodents nearly doubled their lifespan. The extensions varied between species but on average there was a 30–40% increase in lifespan in both mice and rats. Caloric restriction has also been shown to preserve a range of structural and functional parameters in aging rodents.[6]

Activity Levels

Laboratory rodents on a CR diet tend to exhibit increased activity levels at feeding times, particularly when provided with exercise equipment. In one study, animals on a conventional diet showed little activity by early middle age, while those on CR diet were observed to run around the cage and climb onto and hang from the wire tops throughout their lifespan. In fact, the longest surviving CR mouse was observed hanging from the top of his cage only three days before he became moribund.[7] Monkeys on CR diets also appear more restless immediately before and after meals.[8] This is because under a CR diet the subject still get hungry, unlike the pranic lifestyle where the subject is not dependent on physical nourishment.

---

[6] Mattson, Mark P. (2005). "ENERGY INTAKE, MEAL FREQUENCY, AND HEALTH: A Neurobiological Perspective*". Annual Review of Nutrition 25: 237–60.doi:10.1146/annurev.nutr.25.050304.092526.PMID 16011467.

[7] Means, L. W., Higgins, J. L., & Fernandez, T. J. (1993). Mid-life onset of dietary restriction extends life and prolongs cognitive functioning. Physiology & Behavior, 54, 503–508.

[8] Vitousek, K. M., Manke, F. P., Gray, J. A., & Vitousek, M. N. (2004). Caloric Restriction for Longevity: II—The Systematic Neglect of Behavioural and Psychological Outcomes in Animal Research. European Eating Disorders Review, 12(6), 338-360.

Reduced DNA Damage

Calorie restriction reduces the production of reactive oxygen species (ROS)[9] which causes different types of DNA damage such as the presence of 8-hydroxy-2-deoxyguanosine (8-OHdG). These indicators are used to measure the level of oxidative damage in DNA. On CR diets, decreased 8-OHdG damage has been observed in the DNA of hearts, skeletal muscles, brains, livers and kidneys in mice. The levels of 8-OHdG in the organs of 15 month old mice was reduced to 81% of the levels in the DNA of mice on an unrestricted diet.[10] In rats aged 24–26 months on a CR diet, the level of 8-OHdG in the organs was found to be on average 62% of the level in rats fed an unrestricted diet. In mice of the same age, the damage averaged 71% of the level in mice on an unrestricted diet.[11] The scientific explanation is that the body knows how to minimize its energy expenditures, how to reuse, recycle and work more effectively and efficiently and how to use its resources more accurately, and genes alert the body when required.

---

[9] Gredilla R, Sanz A, Lopez-Torres M, Barja G. (2001). Caloric restriction decreases mitochondrial free radical generation at complex I and lowers oxidative damage to mitochondrial DNA in the rat heart. FASEB J 15(9):1589-1591. PMID 11427495 Sohal RS, Ku HH, Agarwal S, Forster MJ, Lal H. (1994). Oxidative damage, mitochondrial oxidant generation and antioxidant defenses during aging and in response to food restriction in the mouse. Mech Ageing Dev 74(1-2):121-133. PMID 7934203

[10] Sohal RS, Agarwal S, Candas M, Forster MJ, Lal H. (1994). Effect of age and caloric restriction on DNA oxidative damage in different tissues of C57BL/6 mice. Mech Ageing Dev 76(2-3):215-224. PMID 7885066

[11] Hamilton ML, Van Remmen H, Drake JA, Yang H, Guo ZM, Kewitt K, Walter CA, Richardson A. (2001). Does oxidative damage to DNA increase with age? Proc Natl Acad Sci U S A 98(18):10469-10474. PMID 11517304

Being breatharian tops caloric restriction because one's body is preserved in a highly clean state at all times. It no longer has to deal with the daily struggle of pushing out toxins. Since there are significantly fewer toxins going into the body, it is easier to fight potential intruders such as viruses and negative bacteria. In short, the body has amazing cleansing powers when it is not preoccupied with the process of digestion. In ideal conditions, each cell works as its own power plant; it consumes energy, cleans itself and excretes the garbage. When we fast, one of the first things the body does is start detoxifying and ridding itself of excess dietary remnants.

Living longer does not have to mean humans have to grow old and become senile. We can continue to lead lives of vitality and good health. Breatharian bodies undergo less stress because energy is not wasted on digestion. This promotes stronger and more efficient use of the internal organs in everyday life. Imagine that for every week you spend on a caloric restricted lifestyle, you get to live an extra two days. *How much is that worth to you?*

To better understand longevity, compare the lifespan of your body to the mileage of a car. A car records mileage, just like the body has a certain lifespan. The car's inner fuel and oil filters can be compared to the body's internal organs—they also record mileage and can only last for so long. A car's filters need to be replaced after a certain time but we have no easy method to replace internal organs when they start to deteriorate with age. This generally means that the more we use our filters, the dirtier they become and our 'car' will not run to its full potential and will not reach the longest mileage it is capable of.

Our bodies take in what they need from food and try to get rid of what they do not need. Due to contemporary changes in our eating habits and decreased availability of quality food, our bodies often do not know how to process or get rid of all the toxins we ingest on a daily basis. Diets based on convenience like processed foods, particularly with added sugar, overthrow the body's natural alkaline balance.

This in turn creates the perfect acidic environment for disease. Furthermore, in the animal kingdom you will notice that humans are the only species on the planet who continue to eat during sickness. Look carefully at nature, look at your pets! When they feel sick, they don't eat! Instead, they allow their bodies to clean themselves through fasting because it encourages healing. Our children have the same instincts, yet it is often with the encouragement of parents that they are taught to ignore this natural reflex. You may notice that when you feel sick, your appetite decreases.

Reduced Toxins

Research also indicates that diseases are usually derived from a build-up of toxins entering the body from modern human diets. Toxins can be small molecules, peptides or proteins capable of causing diseases on contact via the absorption by bodily tissues interacting with biological macromolecules such as enzymes or cellular receptors. Toxins vary greatly in severity.

To be completely free of toxins means you have a much stronger immune system. Most of the toxins that accumulate in the body come from our food in the way it is grown and/or processed. The quantity and quality of food we eat—too many ingredients, large portions, poor food combinations and environmental pollution—can create toxic chemical reactions in the gut. Even if you are eating the best, freshest organic produce, large portions strain the digestive system.

Analyzing data from three national surveys of 60,000 Americans, researchers at the University of North Carolina at Chapel Hill found that serving sizes have grown over the past 20 years. This occurs not only at fast-food outlets but also in restaurants and homes. The data reveals that over the past 20 years the size of hamburgers increased by 23%, a plate of Mexican food is 27% larger, soft drinks grew in size by 52% and snacks like potato chips, pretzels and crackers are 60% bigger.

Not surprisingly, the prevalence of adult obesity in the United States has increased from 14.5% in 1971 to 39.8% in 2016[12]. The problem is that the more you're served, the more you eat. Most people could reduce their meal portion sizes by half and feel an improvement in vitality and energy levels within as little as a week. The problem is that many people are addicted to the sensation of feeling full and do not know when to stop eating before they hit this sensation.

Digesting large quantities of food also takes time and ironically, our digestive systems use a large percentage of the energy stored in the food itself for the digestion process. As already mentioned, when the time spent on digestion is reduced the body has more time to clean itself and recycle energy in a more efficient way.

Of all the food categories, the digestion of proteins is the most time consuming. It takes over three hours to break down and assimilate proteins. The reason for this is simple: protein molecules are long chains with well-soldered links and to break down their resistance requires the combination of good chewing and the simultaneous action of various gastric, pancreatic and biliary juices. This long process of calorie extraction taxes the system.

It has been calculated that to obtain 100 calories from a protein food, the system must use 30 calories. We can say that the specific dynamic action of proteins is 30 percent, while it is only 12 percent for fats and just 7 percent for carbohydrates.[13] The ongoing cycle of the standard three meals per day means a lot of time is spent on digestion and many people need to rest after a meal to aid this process.

----

[12] Prevalence of Obesity Among Adults and Youth: United States, 2015–2016 https://www.cdc.gov/nchs/data/databriefs/db288.pdf

[13] Pierre Dukan, Nutrition & Dietetics, http://www.sharecare.com/question/why-digest-protein-fats-carbohydrates

Almost all of us suffer from occasional constipation or a case of the runs—some more than others. Some of us eat too much too fast until we feel like we are about to explode and must stop. Poor food combinations contribute to discomfort in the stomach. When you take food out of the equation, you liberate yourself from this cycle of discomfort. Breatharians do not need this downtime after dinner or lunch since there is no dinner or lunch! There is simply an abundance of energy not disturbed by the digestion process. There are also no thoughts such as, *Oh, it's noon and I haven't eaten yet.* You are free to need nothing, free from meal times and free to spend your time as you wish.

Breatharians rely on prana—the purest and cleanest source of nourishment available on earth. In fact, it is the original source of life energy on earth. When we eat food, we technically eat prana in its secondary and third forms filtered through the plants and animals we consume.

My own blood tests taken before and after the pranic initiation process showed a significant and stable health improvement. Other breatharians who exit the process and take blood tests show similar improvements. This supports the claim that breatharians do not need to consider the nutritional balance of food or supplement their diets with expensive vitamins. The body gets everything it needs from prana.

Ideal Weight

This is perhaps the most important of all the health benefits which breatharians experience. When living from prana, the body is better able to adjust itself to its ideal weight. Achieving this perfect balance is far more difficult when an individual is distracted by food. I am currently carrying 10% body fat—a percentage that typically only athletes acquire. I am no athlete, although I like to keep in shape. A lower percentage of body fat is connected with a healthier body and ideal weight. In nature, the body of an animal becomes perfectly aligned to its individual needs.

In your mind's eye, try to imagine an obese cheetah in the wild. It is a bizarre, nearly unimaginable image, is it not? Humans have beautiful gifts of self-consciousness and free will to use for better or for worse. Unfortunately, most of us get distracted by food and step out of the perfect balance that nature is able to provide for us.

Body Control

Temperature limits expand for breatharians. This means you can feel comfortable even in extreme hot or cold temperatures. You may also experience increased pain tolerance. In my personal life for example, I sometimes do not notice I am cold because I do not feel cold. I look at my arm and see that I have goose bumps. In hotter temperatures, I am more comfortable and sweat less.

Teeth, Skin and Body Odor

Absence of excess food consumption means no bacterial and food remnants are stored in the body. This also means less dental problems. In my experience, the breatharian process also solved various skin issues such as dandruff and acne. In many cases a person's skin becomes smoother, softer and body odor is significantly reduced.

Feeling 'Light'

Imagine feeling free, energetic and having a good mental attitude from eating well! Breatharians generally feel optimistic and full of energy because, without digestion to stress the body and muddle the mind, daily existence feels clean and pure. This becomes your new emotional baseline and is maintained throughout the day despite the problems or speed bumps life may throw at you. You feel lighter, refreshed and things go smoothly in a positive direction. It's like the feeling after a workout or a good night's sleep, only it stays with you!

Individual Benefits

Knowing that you are living mostly from pure energy dramatically changes your life perspective. You begin to better understand the way the mind works and you can master self-control. You receive a deeper understanding of reality—you realize you are playing a game and in this game you are the creator. It is a game played by consciousness. It is the game of being a human being and the theme of the game is: *you* as you see yourself here in this life. The levels of the game consist of your life experiences, your lessons and your spiritual growth.

A Happier Life

Playing the game as a breatharian allows you to choose how to perceive your life and the life you live becomes what you perceive it to be. Choose happiness and fitness and believe in your own inner strengths. When you understand you are the creator of your own reality, you discover heaven on earth.

A Worthwhile Challenge

Life is full of challenges and this is a gift! Think about it—without challenges there can be no growth. Each challenge teaches us more about ourselves and pushes our limitations and expectations higher and higher. It teaches us patience and self-discipline. It gives us more self-confidence.

Our memory system is directly connected to our senses as well as to our high and low emotional states. You will not remember what you did at 6pm on a normal Tuesday two weeks ago, but you will remember breaking your own bowling record since it is directly connected to a feeling of achievement —an important event. I like the expression, *life is easy for those who live it hard* because I believe one has to endure in order to appreciate. This is why over-spoiling our children can hinder them when they grow older. The feeling of your first hard-earned, money-bought item is better when you know you have worked to achieve it.

The challenge of being a breatharian can be great; some of the difficulties are discussed in a later chapter. Facing the challenges and overcoming them teaches us persistence and strengthens our ability to persevere. This builds strong character. A person who gives up quickly or who changes his or her mind all the time will invariably cope less well with difficulties throughout their lives. If we want to trust ourselves, we need to trust that we will persist when required, give all we can and do our sincere best before we give up.

Appreciation

A breatharian discovers how to truly appreciate sensory input. One learns how to appreciate even the tiniest flavor in a drink. Your sensitivity sensory stimulation is dramatically amplified. Those who go back to eating describe a newfound appreciation for the flavors and textures of food as well as for the endurance of the physical body—the vessel which has amazing abilities and enables us to have great experiences.

Less Sleep and Less Shopping

This is my personal favorite! The basic rule of thumb for a breatharian is that they only need about two thirds of their typical sleeping hours.

The most logical explanation for this is that the body requires less energy to digest food and is therefore less tired. I also have a more complex theory, namely that during sleep our minds sync with higher vibrations and the Higher Self.

As I understand it, breatharians require less sync-time because they are connected to their Higher Selves throughout the waking day. A normal human being either goes to sleep late and wakes up late or goes to sleep early and wakes up early. Research shows that only 4% of the population sleeps for about 3-4 hours a night. I used to envy this four percent; I am now one of them and sleep between three and five hours a night instead of seven to eight hours before my initiation. Sleeping less became a wonderful gift. I started to go to sleep between 1am to 3am and woke up around 6am or 7am to meditate and be the first one in the office (I love my job). As my mornings became longer, I took up frequent meditations and did basic exercises or read a chapter from an inspiring book before starting the day. I started watching movies, took long walks and learned to play the guitar.

All this additional time can be used for spiritual growth, learning and self-fulfillment. It is an opportunity for us to reach higher levels of self-mastery. Another reason for the decreased hours is that I became less preoccupied with food. I did not need to shop often, prepare food or wash the dishes. Shopping is now an occasional event to pick up some juice or basic fresh fruits for a tasty smoothie. This simpler life without feeling thirsty or hungry or needing to nourish myself with food also allows me to seek out exciting new taste experiences.

Financial Independence

Although this is not one of the main considerations you should think about before you become a breatharian, it is true that food is one of our highest living expenses. Whether the food comes from the supermarket, eating out or ordering in, most of our paychecks go toward feeding ourselves.

There are also indirect expenses such as spending money on gas to drive to stores. Saving money in this way makes us less dependent on the currently accepted system and allows us more money to spend on the things that ultimately make us happier as individuals. The key word here is: *independence*.

Not Thinking About Food

Because eating is a daily habit, most of us eat according to the clock. We wake up and eat; it's one o'clock at work, so we eat; we come home from work and we eat. Some of us also have serious issues and a lot of self-judgment around eating. We judge ourselves by what we eat and how much we eat. We find ourselves in a negative or positive emotional state and either console ourselves or celebrate with food.

All of this hinges on our own perceived body image—how we physically look versus the way we think we look and the way we think others think and feel about the way we look. Our personal relationships with food are complicated and hard to define unless considered individually. Whether one is a body builder or a high school student, a tremendous amount of thinking and emotional energy goes into what, when, and how much we eat. As a breatharian, all this is simplified. It is a great advantage not to have to deal with any of this mind-play. These are the basic building blocks of happiness. In addition, if you are overweight before beginning the process, a breatharian lifestyle will ultimately bring you to your ideal weight. For most people, this means they can stop worrying about how they look, forget about diseases that may be incurred because of excess weight and accept that they are at their finest when they are living a breatharian life.

Spiritual Benefits

Long ago when I began my crusade to 'change the world', as some new-agers would call it, I was naive enough to believe I could talk sense into people and I tried to change the ones I met. I have since come to realize that the only way one can truly change things in others as well as the entire world is by setting an inspiring example.

Being a Real Life Example to Others

Becoming a breatharian allowed me to set a personal example for breaking down the illusions that keep us locked into this widely accepted sub-human form. Leading by example can bring about changes in consciousness. It allows me to illustrate to others that we do not really have material needs; we just want stuff, but in the wanting there is beauty.

This is a very liberating insight because it means human beings are able to reach their highest potential and highest levels of happiness. It assists in shattering our myths about want and need and opens our minds to new possibilities.

Happy For No Reason

You do not need anything to be happy, but we live in a society which keeps forgetting that.

I have embraced a *happy for no reason* philosophy since 2007 and completely live this truth. This is a philosophy that destroys dependence on external fantasies to be happy. In other words, you might think a new cell phone, a lover or a good grade at school will make you happy but when you actually achieve these things, more often than not your mind remains unsatisfied. To cope, it instantly seeks the next big distraction. The result? Sustainable happiness remains repetitively elusive.

Furthermore, most people will not allow themselves to be happy without a specific reason to be happy. This sets one up for failure because when you base your happiness on an external reason, the reason can be taken away from you. Your partner might break up with you or you might lose your job, your money or your health. You may also stop appreciating the new car/ cell phone/ apartment that you have.

One of the best ways to retain a high, constant level of happiness is to have no specific reason for happiness. If everything in your life is fine and nothing is severely negative, why not just be happy and content with what you have in the present moment?

Ideally, to maintain personal happiness one should cultivate an attitude of gratitude. Remind yourself daily of all the beauty in your life—the little things and the big things, the relationships you share with friends and family, the comforts you are blessed with, the smells and visual poetry that surrounds you every waking minute in the world.

Secondly, don't take bad things too seriously; everything that arises will eventually pass. Be grateful that you are healthy, that you have people who love you, that you are alive in an amazingly complex body and that you have time for self-realization—otherwise you would not be reading this book! Be grateful that you have options in life, that you have freedom and can exercise free will. There are so many good things we should all be grateful for. If you make a list it will not end quickly and you will find yourself sitting around for a long time with a huge smile.

Mind Over Matter

We all understand mind over matter intuitively but many people fail to grasp the fullness of the fact that there is truly nothing stronger in this world than the human mind. In the process of becoming a breatharian, you prove to yourself that the spirit transcends the physical world and the mind is the key to creating your reality. Furthermore, a breatharian understands the power of faith more than most. Faith or trust means relinquishing your power to greater forces along with your personal belief system — this is what builds your reality.

When you become a breatharian you truly understand that if you can imagine something, it is possible to achieve it. If one does not need food to live, perhaps there is also no need for water. Likewise, perhaps there is no need for us to get sick, age or even[14] die. The power of faith is a big subject with a wide spectrum of possibilities. In some cases, it can cure diseases as discovered with the placebo effect. When you come to understand this fully, your world will change for the better.

Greater Connection To Your Higher Self

Without food there is less matter to keep you grounded on Earth and in human affairs. This amplifies your connection to your Higher Self, the Superego and the astral planes[15]. This is powerful because when our connection to our Higher Self is strong, we feel empowered. We become peaceful, intuitive, knowing and we *feel* more. In this way, we understand the unity of life and our connection with all living beings.

---

[14] I'm currently investigating these subjects and I have even heard of a person who doesn't need to breathe.

[15] The astral planes are considered to be the 'many mansions' described in the Christian Bible. They denote the various realms in spirit that a soul could encounter either after physical death, through a meditation or from an out-of-body experience.

Environmental Benefits

Did you know that it takes between 5,000 and 20,000 liters of water to produce 1 kilogram of beef? This number sounds seriously wrong and inflated, but it is true. This calculation takes into account the entire process beginning with the irrigation of the animal's food crops all the way to how much and what the animal drinks.

Helping Mother Earth

It is not just omnivores who impact negatively on the earth. Did you know that over 30% of the average household garbage bag is filled with compostable bio waste? In addition, there are direct and indirect types of pollution generated by manufacturing plants, the need for numerous watering pipes in these plants and the trucks that move food products.

Eliminating Waste In The Food Industry

The primary areas that require pollution control in the food-processing industry are wastewater and solid waste.

Wastewater

Of concern here are biochemical oxygen demand (BOD) and total suspended solids (TSS) in wastewater which have a negative impact on the receiving environment. The same goes for excessive nutrient loading, namely nitrogen and phosphorous compounds, pathogenic organisms resulting from animal processing and residual chlorine and pesticide levels. BOD measures the amount of food or organic carbons that bacteria can oxidize. The higher the BOD value, the greater the amount of organic matter available for oxygen consuming bacteria. When BOD levels are high, dissolved oxygen (DO) levels decrease; the oxygen available in the water is consumed by bacteria. Less dissolved oxygen in the water means that fish and other aquatic organisms may not survive. In short, high BOD indicates polluted water. This measurement assesses the effect which discharged wastewater has on the environment. TSS indicates the dry-weight of particles trapped by a filter.

It is a water quality parameter that may be used to assess the quality of wastewater after treatment in a wastewater treatment plant.

Solid Waste

Both organic and packaging wastes generated by the food industry need to be processed. Organic wastes are rinds, seeds, skin and bones from raw foods, plus the residue from processing operations. Inorganic wastes typically include excessive packaging materials such as plastics, glass and metal. The good news is that organic wastes are finding ever-increasing markets for resale and companies are slowly switching to more biodegradable and recyclable products for packaging. Excessive packaging is being reduced and recyclable products such as aluminum, glass and high-density polyethylene (HDPE) are used where possible.

Fruit and Vegetable Waste

The wastewater generated by the fruit and vegetable processing industry is high in suspended solids, organic sugars and starches and may contain residual pesticides. For the most part, solid waste not resold as animal feed is handled in conventional biological treatments or composting. The total amount of material generated is a function of the amount of raw material moved through a facility. For example, a given weight of apples produces a given weight of peel and seed waste.

Meat, Poultry and Seafood Waste

Meat, poultry, and seafood facilities produce waste streams that are more difficult to treat than fruit and vegetable wastes. The killing and rendering processes create blood by-products and waste streams extremely high in BOD, the negative effects of which have already been discussed.

These facilities are prone to spreading disease via pathogenic organisms carried and transmitted by the livestock, poultry and the seafood they process. Waste streams vary by facility but can be generalized as process wastewaters such as carcass and skeleton waste, rejected or unsatisfactory animals, fats, oils and greases (FOG), animal faeces and blood and eviscerated organs. Most facilities produce all of these.

The above barely scratches the surface of pollution, misuse and food waste. Just imagine the food chain from the source all the way to your plate. Take into account the trucks used to transport, the packaging, the store that houses the products, supply rooms and staff and you can see that for everything we eat there is a long trail of impurity that impacts on the environment.

When we look objectively at today's processes of food production, we find that it is not done with love and consciousness. Monsanto's[16] worldwide monopoly, now bought out by Bayer, produces chemical wastes that run off into the earth and damages the delicate biodiversity that is needed to make this planet run harmoniously. By becoming a breatharian, you rid yourself of much of the bad karma associated with how your food ends up on your plate.

---

[16] The Monsanto Company was an American agrochemical and agricultural biotechnology corporation that existed from 1901 until it was acquired by Bayer in 2018. It was headquartered in Creve Coeur, Greater St. Louis, Missouri. Monsanto was a leading producer of genetically engineered (GE) seed and Roundup, a glyphosate-based herbicide.

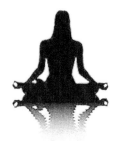

PART TWO

CHAPTER FIVE

My Personal Story

My Pranic Living Process

Knowing that you are going into the breatharian process is a preparation in itself. Even though I wanted to mentally and physically prepare myself for the journey, my guide insisted that everything would happen in the process itself. There was no need for additional pre-process tasks, except of course for the one week raw food diet prior to the process. The raw food diet is not mandatory but helps to release toxins that would otherwise be released during the pranic living process itself and might make the extended process physically easier.

Since I already had a good seven-year practice of a one-day fast on a weekly basis, I already knew what happens to the body during fasting and knew what to expect. The only practice that was necessary for me was a mental one—letting go of my favorite foods plus social expectations and standards. The last thing for me to do was train myself to be judged and perhaps ridiculed from time to time because of my choice. Since breatharians are mostly unknown in the western world, I knew most of the difficulties after the process would most likely be social. I expected full support from my wonderful, supporting, semi-hippy family but some of my friends were a different matter altogether.

To best prepare myself, I did everything I needed to close the open issues in my life as if I was going for a long jungle vacation. It came at a perfect time since the start-up company I was working for had been bought by another company.

During the in-between time of the acquisition, I could take the liberty of a long vacation. I rented out my Tel-Aviv apartment, paid all my bills, left an auto-alert message on my email and let the important people in my life know that I would absolutely not be available for the following three weeks.

Since I did not know what the outcome of the process would be, I decided not to tell everyone where I was going. Most of my inner circle was not aware that this life option was real and so I wanted to let them know about the process only after I went through it. This was to ensure that their negative remarks would not influence me and affect my subconscious mind during the three weeks. I decided to tell those closest to me where I was going. I spoke to my partner at the time, my parents and my sister who was to be my caretaker (a role which is described in Chapter 7—How to Become a Breatharian). It was important to tell them that after the process my body would take time to recover and that I would return quite skinny. It was important for me to prepare them for my own journey as I would require their understanding, or rather, lack of judgment.

I was driven to my selected location and unpacked the many things I thought would be important during my time there. The process itself began at midnight, so my spouse had time to say goodbye and spend some time at the location with me.

For my last meal, I decided to have a persimmon. I remember I took just one bite of it and immediately realised it must have gone bad. I spit it out and understood that my lesson was a lesson in absolute release from solid food. I was happy that the fruit had gone bad—it was one less thing to think about.

I could write an entire book about what happened during the pranic living process. The personal journal I wrote at the time is on my website. Those of you who are interested can use Google to translate the passages as many have already done. I attempt to provide the best highlights from the journal here.

The first three days of the process are days of cleansing. This cleansing and detoxification are done automatically by the body. Since I did not allow myself any water in the first week, my body had to use its supplies by taking water from my muscles, organs and fat. Remember, this is a process so in the beginning it is just a long dry fast.

The cleansing was both emotional and physical. Water, as many new researchers have documented, contains information. Our toxins and emotional states are saved inside the water in our body. This is why a dry last is excellent for releasing and cleaning both the body and mind.

The body is using up its old batteries and energy sources, forcing itself to break apart old cells that are no longer at their energetic prime. In addition, water is finally being brought out of the darkest areas of the body and while the body resets itself to be more energy efficient, it lowers the blood pressure to save energy.

Since there were absolutely no normal things to be done throughout the process, I started developing my own schedule. I had a drawing board and a lot of art to make, especially sacred geometry, painting and puzzles. I tried to get into the habit of doing stretches every day.

Each sunrise and sunset I spent time outside gazing at the sun and meditating on it. I read an average of half a book a day. Most books were on spiritual or scientific topics. I followed my intuition. It whispered to me that the knowledge I was obtaining during the process would be integrated deep within my subconscious.

During the first three days I felt like I was actually just waiting and building a happy state of being for the rest of the process. These are days of belief, of fasting and of acknowledging what it is you are concentrating on to accomplish. Many define these days as the days of small amounts of doubt. This is because you have not yet had the one hundred percent assurance in your abilities. Starting on the night of the third day something special started to happen.

If you read the 21-day guidelines in the book *Pranic Nourishment—Living on Light* by Jasmuheen, you will understand that you are actually reactivating ancient knowledge we used to have but lost. To achieve this state of awareness one must from the fourth day on, incorporate three intervals of two hours each during which time it is recommended that you do not move but lie down in the same position.

The intervals can get boring—after all, it is a 6-hour meditation on a daily basis. The purpose of the intervals is to allow contract holders and process observers to work on your body, fix energy tunnels and detoxify and balance the four bodies. I was quite amazed by the sensations that went through my body. It was the first time that I felt another presence 'touching' me. I felt wavy energy all over the right side of my face which I could influence and control with meditation and breathing. I also felt a concentration of energy shifting wherever I had a scar on my body. It was as if the energy that had been stuck in that spot was released and was able to start flowing freely. Since then I have heard many different accounts of physical sensations experienced by people who have completed the process with me as their guide. These four crucial days are what I call *the surgery* and are the highlight of the process. After the four days we continue in *recovery*, allowing the body time to integrate the new, or should I say, *ancient and forgotte*n technology and beliefs into itself.

When the seventh day finally arrived, I was relieved. My guide had physically come for the first and only time during the process for my first water drink. The water ceremony is short and exciting. I read a small prayer and acknowledged water as purifying and mesmerizing and allowed it into my body for the first time in my new life. Imagine being without water for an entire week. During that week you are not allowed to swallow any water at all, not even a drop. I took showers and brushed my teeth but only held water in my mouth. Not drinking even a drop is crucial for the success of the process.

Without water one fears dehydration, especially during such an extended period of time, but nothing bad happens to those who believe in the process. I remember clearly that during the third and fourth day I became weaker, mostly due to lower blood pressure. This caused some minor dizziness from time to time especially when I stood up too quickly.

Lacking water had a great psychological effect on me. I missed it a lot and I learned how to appreciate this fine element from an entirely different point of view. Even my subconscious missed it so much that it became the subject of many dreams I had at the time. In some dreams, I watched a glass of water continuously elude my grasp while in other dreams I just felt a deep need to drink.

However, I was really surprised that I did not get thirsty at all. The only thing I physically felt being in that state was that my throat was always dry. It is a constant reminder that you are in the process and it never goes away during the first week. Even when I washed my mouth with water, I only had half a minute of relief and then my throat went quickly back to being completely dry. Amazingly enough, throughout the week I continued to pass urine. It was dark and orange and had a strong odor. The first few days the color and smell was strong, but after that it became pure and watery. I understood that the kidneys continue to clean the body even when the body is not taking in any new water.

After my first glass of water, I felt naturally high. I stopped meditating and deviated from my daily schedule on purpose. I had come to the realization that anything I did during the process was automatically in a meditative state, so no intentional meditations were required. Time had shifted for me and I seemed to have more time to actually be in the present moment in whatever I decided to do. I took pleasure in almost everything. I took much longer to enjoy stretching, showering or gazing at the sky or smelling a flower. On one occasion, I even followed an ant and some of her friends for a few hours! It was an incredible sensation of oneness with all that is.

The days turned into nights and I slowly forgot about the outside world while the process intensified. I only talked to my caretaker and my guide once a day and these were ten minute conversations each. I had not yet missed the outside world and I was incredibly happy in my isolation.

The second and third weeks were easier than the first. My guide had given me some exercises and meditations; some were contemplations about mindfulness, gratitude and forgiveness. Some were mind games to keep me and my mind busy while others were meant to assist me in shifting my consciousness to a higher state of being and to release parts of my education and my past. I will refrain from describing the actual exercises and meditations as they are kept secret for those who choose to become breatharians. I will say that I enjoyed all of them and each had a specific goal, whether to clear the mind, to shift one's understanding about the world or to simply let go of parts of the past that are no longer necessary to hold on to.

The third week is defined as the *integration* week and it is the first time that you can start leaving your habitat. I started walking a little more each day until I was walking five to six kilometers per day towards the end. I had more and more energy with each passing day. Other sensations also started changing. Since I did the process in the middle of January, it was winter and cold outside. During my short hikes I found that my body behaved differently. I started walking more upright, my mind felt clearer and sharper and I felt more in control, more vivid and more aware of myself.

Allow me to elaborate using the body temperature as an example. Before the process I had normal sensations of cold and warm but now I felt as if my body was allowing me less negative sensations. This means I still understood that my body was cold but it was as if I was watching it from the outside and witnessed the *symptoms* of being cold instead of experiencing the *sensation* of being cold. It was as if I had been given control over my internal temperature.

The same happened to me with pain. It felt that my pain tolerance increased overnight. Even though there is plenty more to say about what happened in my process and the changes that happened during and after it, I have decided not to elaborate more on it at this time. Perhaps one day I will have my personal journal translated and edited and will release it for a deeper understanding of this hidden, but most important and interesting process. Until then, as previously mentioned, it is available on my website.

Preparations For My Initiation

Four months after first hearing about breatharianism I contemplated undergoing the process myself, sometimes I even had dreams about what it would be like. I also talked to as many people as possible who had experienced the process first-hand to assure myself that I was ready for it and to find out what I could expect to happen. Then one day I abruptly decided to go for it. Thinking about and understanding this lifestyle is one thing; I wanted to really know it and feel it with my own body. Besides that, I have always loved a good challenge and I was never very good at cooking.

The day you decide to set the date for your process is the day you actually start your process.

I decided to set my date for mid-January 2013. I chose this date because it continued on from the 21st of December 2012. That date, according to some, held a significant shift in the earth's energy fields and it was believed that great changes would occur. It was also known as the end of the Maya's historical calendar and the end of a few major earth cycles. I had been researching this auspicious 21st of December 2012 date for many years, as it signified a change in the frequency of our collective consciousness. Of course I was expecting something big to happen, yet the day came and went without event. Later, I realized that this 'something big' was up to me and so I decided to become a breatharian.

My own preparations for the process brought me face-to-face with some of my fears—the first of which was a week-long dry fast without water. Science tells us that a person is likely to die after four days without water.

To overcome this, I decided to test the water a little before diving in, so to speak. I undertook an air fast for a few days whilst maintaining my own routine of working and exercising. That went rather smoothly and I was happy to find out that it wasn't as difficult as I had anticipated.

Another exercise I did was to slowly let go of my favorite foods when I went shopping. This is by no means a mandatory exercise but I wanted to experience the loss of certain tastes to see how I would cope. I released one flavor at a time from my diet before the 'big bang'.

The first thing I stopped buying was cheese. Okay, so I would still allow myself pizza and other cheesy foods when I went out with my friends or when I really wanted them but it was no longer a routine item I kept in my fridge. Over the course of two months pending my process, I began to slowly relinquish my attachment to other favorite foods.

Setting the date was one thing but I also had some organizing to do to ensure the process would run smoothly. This included finding a suitable location for the process, subletting my apartment and organizing leave from work so that the rest of my world was ready for my three-week long absence.

I also had to appoint a caretaker to look after me during the process. This was a position my sister was happy to fill. Most people do not get to have a family member as a caretaker. Most parents and siblings get scared when a family member embarks on this process. They worry, thinking the person has lost their grip on reality in a 'new age' experiment. I was lucky enough to have my sister's support from the start.

Tal naturally became my breatharian guide and we met a few times before the process to ensure that I was mentally ready and that I was doing it for the right reasons.

It was during our last meeting in Tel-Aviv right before my ride came to take me to my 21-day location, that Tal told me something I will never forget. He said, "What you are about to do is not taken for granted. I am proud of you." It wasn't until he spoke these words that I truly began to feel the fullness of my commitment. As his words echoed in my ears, I asked myself one last time, *Am I really going to stop eating?*

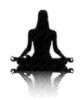

Post-Process Life

Life just is not the same after a pranic initiation. You cannot ignore the changes that occur both internally and externally throughout the process. Your behavior is different, your perspective is different and perhaps even your character is different. Of course, you are who you always were but it is easier to express yourself. In a nutshell, there is less ego and more soul.

I can split my life after the process in two: mental changes and sensory changes. I came to fully understand that living from light was no longer just a theory. I was walking the streets of Tel-Aviv with boundless energy. I was amazed at the capacity of the human body. I was smiling, feeling high and on top of the world. Life was once again exciting and new after the process.

Even simply seeing strangers on the street was different. I suddenly had an urge to explain to them everything about what I had discovered. I wanted to explain to them that we are not just our physical bodies—that we are in fact so much more than that! I wanted to explain this newfound connection to spirit; that *we are spiritual beings in search of a human experience— not the other way around* and that we can transcend almost anything. I could now clearly see how our physical body becomes a part of a very complicated, self-created illusion. Sadly, most people were not ready to hear these things from me.

Nonetheless, a remarkable feeling of self-discovery came with this sensation of achievement and I was radiatiant. It all felt so good, so right.

Over the next few months I also rediscovered my body from another perspective. I soon learned that these months were critical; I was still shifting my consciousness after the process. My prana-percentage was high but in no way perfect. My body was still learning how to thrive on prana and I was still losing weight. For my own sanity, I found myself re-examining my faith.

Post-process I was also feeling many different sensations in my body. Right after the process I was very weak and I knew that it would take some time for me to get back into shape but I wanted to begin immediately. Now, I am not an athlete, but I like to stay in shape by exercising on the beach a few times a week. I also like to take long walks and play with poi.[17] The first few times I exercised were the hardest. I found myself exhausted after only 15 minutes of activity. In addition, walking upstairs either to my apartment or to my office made me really feel my muscles working.

My teeth became more sensitive to hot and cold drinks and I became much more enthusiastic about sweet drinks. In fact, my whole taste experience changed and it continues to change! I tend to fixate on one particular taste at a time for several weeks. In the beginning I only wanted sweet drinks, mostly synthetic, tasty ones. I did not care too much about what went into my mouth since I figured it did not really matter anymore. I got whatever I needed from pranic nourishment. About two and a half months after the beginning of my process, my body stopped losing weight and I have since reached a new balance. I was happy to reach this point rather quickly in comparison to my friends and the experiences I read about which were documented in other pranic books.

---

[17] A type of juggling play that you can also do as a fire performer.

Less than three months is an amazing time in which to achieve this balance! It allowed me to overcome one of the biggest challenges in undergoing the process—looking like a walking skeleton (see Figure 2 below). I continued to gain weight over the course of another 2-3 weeks until I reached the weight that I am at now which is about two kilos under what I used to be. This is ultimately what I consider to be my ideal weight. Soon enough, exercising became as easy as before the process and I went back to my exact weight and exercise timings. I actually find that I have more energy and occasionally want to exercise twice a day.

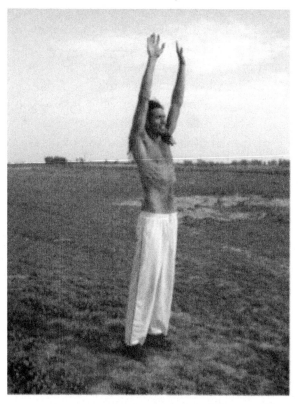

Fig 2. A picture of me taken after my breatharian initiation

Taste

When a person eats regularly, they rarely think about a time when they will not eat or how much they would miss taste. Taste is such an amazing sense that we need to appreciate and give it the respect it deserves. Too many people eat without paying much attention, often focusing on the next bite before even finishing what they have in their mouths. Research shows that after about the third mouthful of food, we stop tasting. Autopilot kicks in and most of us continue to chew until our plates are empty.

Being a breatharian has taught me to appreciate taste differently. Since one of my game rules at the time (see Chapter 12—The Rules of Your Game) was to only take liquids, I allowed myself to bend the rules by taking in things that could melt in my mouth, like chocolate or ice cream. In such instances, I closed my eyes and allowed my senses to take over.

In the past, if I bought a drink and it was not very good, I would still drink it thinking that I spent good money on it and that it served a kind of a purpose in providing me with liquid nutrition. Today, I would just throw it in the garbage. If it does not provide me with a good tasting experience, it is not worth anything to me. I also take my time and try not to drink too fast so that my taste experience can last longer. I use a straw and ensure that every sip counts. I also overheat my tea so it will take longer to drink. I choose what I drink carefully and only drink what I want and what tastes good to me. I use a wine glass to drink a shake because I want to give even the simplest of drinks its well-deserved honor and give myself a sensation of being a king.

It seems that most breatharians tend to develop a sweet tooth. One of the reasons is that it does not really bother them when they eat something that is full of sugar, like ice cream or chocolate. They know they get fed from another source. The other reason is that the body makes everything taste so much better! So your inner child is calling out, "I want sugar!"

Water

My relationship with water has also completely changed. Even though I appreciate water a lot, it has no taste to me. Before my process I used to drink the recommended two liters of water each day. I carried a bottle of mineral water everywhere. Today I hardly drink any water. Why? I stopped believing in the two-liter rule. I understand deeply that it was just a part of the illusion. During the process, especially after the fourth day of dry fasting, I kept passing urine even when I wasn't drinking anything and the color of the urine drastically changed from dark orange to lighter. Something in the mechanism of being a breatharian allows us to not need so much water to live.

Now I will take water only if there is nothing else around for me to have. I will drink a little water to wash my mouth or if I feel that it is a warm day outside and I want some refreshment. Since I no longer have any sensation of thirst and since I did not choose to be a rare[18] breatharian who has stopped drinking water, I still take care of my physical body. I sometimes check my boundaries to see how little water I can take. I once walked three days in the desert and only drank one liter of water a day, when it is recommended to drink between four to five liters a day under those circumstances. My urine was orange, but I felt great and did not have any difficulty or feel dehydrated.

My relationship with water is yet to be concluded. I feel that someday in the future I would like to take the challenge of stopping water for at least one month to test myself. I would like to know if I can do it and what it will feel like. I used to think that food grounds me but now I know that water also grounds a person. The sensation of being on an air fast is slightly 'higher' than being on a water fast. The sensations of cleanliness and connection to the divine are faster and stronger.

---

[18] Currently only 2 breatharians in the world are known to me to have completely stopped drinking water.

Relationships

Coming out of the process, I had a deeper connection with my feminine side. This made me feel complete in many ways. It is important to understand that within each of us there are masculine and feminine energies. The key to living in harmony with one's self is to embrace both sides in proportionate balance with your sexuality. Ideally, the balance of these energies is like yin and yang—a balanced man will have a dominant masculine essence while retaining intuitive feminine qualities and vice versa for women.[19] When these energies thrive in harmony we become complete human beings. However, today's society does not exemplify many balanced role models. This has created much confusion and separation between the sexes, causing people to look externally to the opposite sex for completion.

I was in a relationship when I entered the 21-day process and during that time I had many moments in which to contemplate my relationship. On the one hand, I was in love and I missed my girlfriend a lot. I really wanted to see her and let her know what I was going through. I had also started to plan so many cool and exciting things for us to do together after my return and was looking forward to feeling her in my arms again.

When I finished the process, I realized I had changed. Important aspects of our relationship were not working for the new Ray. It took just a few weeks to go our separate ways once I discovered my new self. This was a blessing, as I needed time alone in the world to understand the new me. Being alone provided a new balance in my feminine and masculine sides and I became gentler and less motivated by ego. My intentions became clearer and I had less dependence on women to feel loved, opening me up to sharing love with all creation.

---

[19] A balanced woman will have dominant feminine energy with masculine qualities like assertiveness, goal directed and independence.

When I had just finished the process, my libido was also low. Yet I felt complete and therefore wasn't looking for external happiness outside my own unity. Physical factors such as still feeling weak and having lower blood pressure contributed to not wanting to have sex or masturbate. Three months later, my libido returned to normal. This was around the time when I also regained weight and my fitness levels started to improve.

Interestingly, there was a big change in the type of woman I now became interested in. I became less concerned about external looks and started looking for a more spiritually aware person. I found that lying was difficult for me and I had a natural desire to be my natural self living my own truth, while respecting the 'whole-package deal', boundaries and free will of the person with whom I would become involved. I find that I can no longer think about meaningless sex or a superficial one-night stand. These days for me it is all about deep connection.

However, with these benefits some challenges also arose. Imagine that you are going out with a guy who does not eat—there are no 'dinner-and-movie' dates. My cupboards are sometimes embarrassingly empty when guests come over. At least now they know not to expect anything from me! There is much less socializing around food, which for many people is an important aspect of being in a relationship. It also means having to provide constant explanations and to endure over-concerned judgments and misunderstandings from friends and family who live differently.

That being said, do not give up hope too soon if you choose to go through this process. While at first you may find the new distance between yourself and others a little challenging as your personal frequency changes, more interesting and understanding people will come into your life. For instance, I recently had a relationship with a girl who was very supportive of my breatharian way of life. The bottom line is this: do you want to be in a relationship with someone who is inspired and supportive of your choices, or threatened and confronted by your commitment to pursuing your fullest potential?

In this way, breatharianism becomes a great filter for attracting partners who are open-minded, spiritually aware and accepting of you as a whole-package deal. After all, in order to have a truly satisfying relationship we need partners who are willing to help us grow and genuinely wish for us to succeed in all our endeavors.

People and Society

For the first few months after the process, you will continuously think about your new way of life. Most people only have an inkling of the extent to which food is embedded into our daily lives. You will find constant reminders and perhaps even temptations reminding you of your choice not to eat. Cities are centered around restaurants, diners, cafes and supermarkets. Wherever you go you see people eating; walking and eating, driving and eating, cooking and eating. Smells saturate your senses.

People may also get curious and inquire about your new extra-skinny physical appearance. Depending on how you choose to react, you will often have to deal with misunderstandings, ridicule and a general lack of belief. In the new Pranic Living Group Initiation, this phase is very small as the new breathing exercises help to restore weight balance much faster.

Socializing becomes a different game and you may begin to perceive it from another perspective. You have changed but the world as a whole has not. As you realize this, you discover new social boundaries with regard to how much of your lifestyle you share with others. Some people will be genuinely curious, others will want to argue with you. This is why many breatharians choose to remain anonymous.

You may also encounter awkward situations where a generous host will offer you food saying, "You have got to taste this pie, I made it myself!" It is important to develop your own way of dealing with situations like these.

Some breatharians will say that they do not eat sugar or give another excuse not to accept the offer. Others will occasionally eat a small portion to avoid giving an explanation or offending a host. Personally, I find that the best way is to say that I am fasting. This is partially true and fasting is becoming more accepted these days by the general population.

Dealing with social rules and standards is usually your biggest challenge. You may feel left out of some situations and have to work a bit harder to break through this illusion. Some friends who know I am a breatharian still continue to offer me food out of politeness or habit. To many people, breatharianism is so rare and strange that it just does not make sense, which means they don't know or forget how to interact with people who practice it.

Some people also do not feel comfortable when they are eating next to me. They ask me time after time if it is okay for them to eat something around me. I find it funny and I take the time to reassure them I have no judgment on their choices. In fact, I love the challenge it brings me and the smell of food around me, so I appreciate it when people eat next to me. It is only during the moments when everybody is eating and the conversation lulls that I feel a little left out.

After about a year into my breatharian experience, I decided to go back to eating a meal once in a while. The first year was amazing but I experienced social difficulties and I no longer needed to prove anything to myself. The shift was amazing and retuning to the taste of solid food was incredible. These days I balance myself with two or three meals a week and some snacks if I feel like it, though I don't need them. There is no more self-judgment on the subject and I feel that I can easily enjoy both worlds.

Why Me?

The question, *Why me?* is actually the question, *Why should I be the one to try and get the word out?* There are hundreds of other breatharians who can do it but it seems that they are not interested in sharing it very much or have simply been burnt by ridicule and misunderstanding.

I have asked myself this question many times. In the beginning I found no answer but after awhile I understood that I am not a typical breatharian. I come from a scientific world. My father is a physicist and researcher. I myself learned and mastered scientific concepts before I chose to combine them with a new spiritual way of life. I think this is what distinguishes me from others; this is my balance. I am a seeking person of extremes who pursues adventures and challenges in everything. Even though most people think science and spirit occupy opposite corners of the room, I see them as one beautifully aligned truth that will in the future, become our new way of understanding that our life on earth is an illusion.

I am both right-brain oriented (intuition, emotion, creativity) and left-brain oriented (logic, memory, thinking). One of the many reasons I went into my breatharian experience was to understand it from a logical point of view even when there is not always a way to do so. I do not seek money or fame through speaking about breatharianism. I do however, feel a great urge to share knowledge that will allow others to open their minds to the infinite possibilities which our illusion allows us.

Understanding that a man does not require food to survive or requires a ridiculously small amount of food, opens us up to an understanding of what and who we truly are. It shows us the triumph of human consciousness over physical reality and makes us second-guess ourselves. The truth I have come to understand is not something that I will share here. I can only say the greater truth is far more complicated than any of us can imagine. Being a breatharian opens you up to accepting more possibilities. Information can be found in science, philosophy and in ancient history but the greater Truth can only be found within us and in our intuition. God, the Prime Creator[20] as I see it, is present in each of us. Like the seed of a tree that contains all the information of the tree in order for it to grow, one human cell contains all the DNA required to duplicate a human body. We *are* the essence, the seed of God. God has created man in his own image. We are God and God is us; it is not an external reality. We are all together God in a godly experience. We are the One in the One's path of expression. There are many explanations I could add here but I want to focus on breatharianism in this book.

My reasons for wanting to get the word out are: to open minds, to communicate with those who seek to know that this lifestyle is a possibility, to make us question what we have been taught by the world about who we are as humans and to make us understand our inner strength and the true power we have as sentient beings. For me, being a breatharian is a part of my search for living a higher truth. I am also a seeker of excitement and challenges. I enjoy it when things get rough, so not having some flavor in my life is not that big a deal. When I really think about it, the experience of flavor disappears after a few minutes while the gifts of the breatharian way of life remain.

---

[20] I call him Prime Creator because I liked this definition from the Pleiadians Awakening Message. There are many creators in the hierarchy.

I question my life choices and my ideals frequently so that I can always remain objective and never allow myself to think that I know something absolutely. Everything changes including scientific discoveries and my own character and will. One of the thoughts that crosses my mind when I think about these life choices is, *What would I do if God had given me a choice before I was born?* The first choice would be a life containing a variety of foods and in that life, I would use my sense of taste more than my other senses. However, that life would have a short lifespan. The possibility of having diseases, less time for other activities and a weaker connection with the divine would be the norm. The second life choice would be the opposite of the first. I would have to give up my dependency on food and miss out on many flavors and textures. However, I would live a longer and healthier life, I would have 20% more time, sleep less, be almost disease and toxin free and have a stronger connection with the divine. Which one would you chose?

I want us to question our lives to find the amazing, all-knowing spirit inside us and never forget that our eyes are temporarily covered from the Absolute Truth by the illusion we find ourselves in. We have chosen to forget but our ultimate goal is to remember. So, let us all wake up, my brothers and sisters!

CHAPTER SIX

The TV Exposure

Lockdown For Eight Days

In September 2013 I was invited to go on a well-known Israeli investigative reporting show. The researchers had found me while investigating alternative nourishment methods via the Internet and had watched a few of my online lectures. At the time, I had an inner knowing that I would soon appear on a public platform for the world to see as a way to spread the word about my lifestyle. There were only two 'serious' breatharians in Israel at the time: my guide and myself. My guide was a very spiritual man and exposing this delicate subject to the mainstream required someone somewhere between the spiritual and scientific worlds. I was the perfect candidate for the job. By conventional standards, I was considered as 'normal' as one could be. The objections people could have had on the subject would not have been about my abnormality. Anyone exposed to the subject would have to search within for their own understanding and answers. For my part, I felt it was a great responsibility and honor to be the one to represent this subject to a wide audience, especially because of the many previous misunderstandings I encountered when I talked to people who had never heard of breatharianism before.

The show is on my website: raymaor.com. I recommend you watch it so you understand a little more about society's amazement with the breatharian lifestyle. The website also contains other video links and information.

Preparing For The Show

Prior to the experiment, the team and I spent a few months planning the logistics and the set-up required by the crew and myself. This included finding a proper location close enough so they could visit me on a daily basis. We found a doctor who would perform surveillance and manage the scientific aspects of the experiment and who took care of a few other less important logistical matters. I told the television crew that I was not 100% breatharian, that I did not wish to be and that I still drank. (There are only two in the world at this time who only live on air.) Most breatharians are like me and we drink or eat small quantities out of choice, *not necessity*.

I explained to them that I was going to lose weight due to not drinking but unlike a person who has not gone through the spiritual process, I would not suffer weakness, dizziness, headaches, dehydration or any other expected symptoms, nor would I become hungry or thirsty. The message was understood and the preparations continued. I told them the only thing that would probably bother me was being harassed by continuous interviews and blood tests. Blood tests have always been an issue for me. Draining my blood makes me feel incomplete like someone is disturbing my energetic field by taking something out of it. I usually have issues like feeling weak or fainting when someone gives me a simple blood test.

There was a third party to the experiment—a wealthy businessman who had started an Internet chat with me a few months prior. He declared that breatharians simply cannot exist and we arranged a one-sided wager of $100,000 USD to see if I could undergo the experiment successfully.

At the time, I did not think about the TV people approaching me, so I did not take the bet too seriously. After all, it was only a guy on a Facebook chat trying to tease me.

Lucky for me, a good lawyer friend pushed me into checking it out. I decided to meet him to show him I'm a real person and not some fake identity behind an Internet wall. We agreed we would conduct a real experiment including scientific research with an objective doctor and that it would be documented by a serious television show. At the time, none of it seemed to have any likelihood of manifesting.

As a student of manifestation and having a deeper understanding of how life and our consciousness correspond with one another, I placed many positive intentions into the experiment. To that I added unselfish reasons of raising global consciousness. I persuaded myself that life would show me the course that would eventually lead me to the prize—not because I deserved it or because of greed, but because I somehow knew both the exposure and the prize were in my life's path.

A normal person does not place such a serious bet for no reason and out of nowhere. I still do not truly understand why the businessman placed that bet. Nevertheless, we signed a legal document two days before the experiment outlining the definition of its success.

The criteria was that I would survive, that the composition of my blood would not change and be confirmed by doctors, that I would not suffer any dehydration symptoms and that my mental and physical condition would be sound.

In addition, we decided on making the experiment eight full days without food *or water*, which I was not accustomed to. As you can probably imagine, finding a doctor who was willing to take part in the experiment was an issue.

All the doctors we interviewed said that what I was going to do was impossible and probably life threatening. They were not prepared to participate in the experiment for fear of their licenses being revoked for non-humanitarian practices.

The first doctor who was willing to participate received a notice from his medical association stating they did not approve of his participation. He immediately and without hesitation resigned from the experiment. We went through a few more candidates until we ended up with a well-known senior cardiologist from a main hospital in Tel-Aviv and he stayed on with us until the end of the experiment.

Even though I lived on a few hundred calories a day at the time and even though I had already done a seven-day dry fast by myself, I did not want to take any chances. Representing something as significant as pranic energy to the public for the first time was something completely new and I wanted it to be as perfect as possible. I felt a big responsibility being the one to carry it out. For months I knew that I was the one who was supposed to bring the pranic living process to the public. I felt it coming ahead of time.

To make sure that all went extra smooth, I decided to have pranic 'workouts'. Every week I had a two-day dry fast without resting—meaning I had my normal schedule of working out, going to my job, making love and other things a normal person does without consideration of what I consumed. I wanted to make sure that my body would raise my pranic intake to its maximum potential. I know that it sometimes takes the body a while to get used to living off prana so in order for the process to go smoothly, it was better to do so ahead of the time rather than worry about doing it all during the experiment.

I only slept about four hours each night and woke up naturally with an abundance of energy. In addition, I felt excited knowing something great was about to happen.

I adopted sunset sun-gazing and Falon Gong[21] exercises. It was a very energetic time for me.

Even though I knew that I would have no problem doing this long dry fast, there were a few unknown factors. The main one was how I would deal with the stress, the constant provocations and interviews, the pressure of appearing in front of hundreds of thousands of people and the potentially materialistic significance of winning a hundred thousand dollars. Dealing with different emotional pressures alone can cause unknown outcomes, especially when you are a breatharian. Any emotion can create unknown consequences as your emotional body becomes out of balance with the rest of the bodies—the physical, spiritual and mental. The second factor was the blood tests. Apart from my personal discomfort, no one is supposed to do blood tests during a dry fast as it torments the body and reduces the amount of liquids in the body. In addition, the doctors did not only want one blood test, they wanted them on a daily basis!

Apart from those two issues, I felt great. I even felt an inner guidance that my spirit wanted me to do the show. Too many good things were happening in sync for me to ignore them. I felt like I was getting assistance from above, so I did not really have anything to worry about. I trusted the universe and I felt obligated to myself and to my fellow human beings to bring more ancient understandings and knowledge out of the closet.

I had several motivations—some egoistic and others altruistic. Simply put, the money was for myself and to raise global consciousness and awareness of our unique abilities. I am both spiritual and materialistic and I found my own balance in that. I am not ashamed to say I was interested in the money.

---

[21] Falun Gong is a Chinese spiritual practice that combines meditation and qigong exercises with a moral philosophy centered on the tenets of truthfulness, compassion and forbearance.

However, I can say the money was not the goal. It was a bonus that came with the experiment. A few days before the experiment, the businessman did not want to go through with it and the producers asked me if we should continue our preparations.

I told them clearly that the bet was not the reason we were doing it and we should continue with or without the third party. Luckily for me, the businessman changed his mind at the last minute. I still don't know why he did what he did. An idea has come to my mind from a higher perspective that the money was used to make a stronger impression on the public, who are still mainly materialistic in this day and age. I understood more people would take the subject seriously if they knew an unknown contributor took it seriously enough to fund a scientific study and bet a large amount of his own cash on it.

Another thought was that I would eventually invest some of this money in the greater good. I live in a world of abundance and therefore I have invested a large part of the prize money into the development of two free energy devices that will benefit the rest of us when the time comes.

The Show

During the show I was monitored by eight cameras and living in a bungalow rented by the production crew for the purpose of constant observation. I was not allowed to leave the general area of the bungalow. The eight cameras were around and within the bungalow which meant that I was monitored by at least one camera at any given time. The cameras visibility boundaries were shown so I could know my boundaries when I stepped outside. I also had a camera in the shower, in the toilet and in the bedroom.

The rules were simple: I was not to eat or drink for eight complete days. I was not allowed to put my head under the water in the shower or wash myself above the neck at all. I was to always be visible through the cameras, to sleep with the lights on and I could not step away from my marked limited area which included the bungalow and its very close surroundings. Every day I was to provide the designated doctor my blood for testing and diagnosis, perform some basic motor function tests and give a urine sample.

When I brushed my teeth I used a marker to draw a horizontal line on a water glass and filled the water up to the line before I washed my mouth. I then spit the water back into the cup when I finished brushing my teeth. I displayed the water glass to the camera before and after to prove that I had not swallowed any water during the mouthwash.

Prior to the experiment the television crew documented several interviews with specialist doctors about the expected results of the experiment. Based on their expertise, they expected me to last for three days before giving up. One of them expected to take me out by force on a stretcher four days in. They predicted that I would be seriously dehydrated, have a dry tongue and have serious and problematic blood tests—mostly in electrolyte count, urea, Hb, haematocrit, WBC and more. They also said that I was risking my life and that my internal organs would not be able to handle the pressure.

The first three days of the experiment were the easiest for me. I wasn't bored yet and my motivation was running high. The process has never been about physical weakness but about my mental attitude. Having previously done the 21-day process, I came prepared and had a good idea of how I was planning to spend my time. Unlike the challenging 21-day process, here I could have access to the outside world. I took my laptop on which I pre-downloaded documentaries and had my cell phone with me at all times. In addition, I was allowed to have a friend come by if I wanted. I only used that option twice because I had a fixed schedule to keep me busy. Every day I woke up and did some Falon Gong exercises to get more energy flowing through my system first thing in the morning. Every sunrise and sunset I did about twenty minutes of sun-gazing followed by a half hour meditation. After that I retreated and did some artwork, drawing mandalas, making small copper trees or other creative work. During the day I watched a movie or a series, did plenty of meditation and listened to online lectures.

Almost every night I had two appointments. The first was with the skeptical doctor who came to test my blood and try to talk me out of the experiment. The second was the television host who always attempted to create some drama to raise viewer interest. I liked both occasions because it made my days more interesting, but I was also very grateful when it ended and I knew I had the night to myself.

After the fourth day, I suddenly started getting really appreciated and respected by the show host. Neither he nor the doctor thought I would ever make it this far and they started realizing that something special was going on. The doctor immediately started speculating on his own terms and worldview about how this could be possible. He wasn't happy that the blood composition did not change over time and that no great physical changes had taken place in my body as he had predicted. In his praise, I must state that he accepted the situation with scientific objectivity and did not try to explain or change his initial opinion.

From the fourth day onward everything went smoothly until the end of the experiment. I continued to have daily visits from the doctor who ran tests and took blood and urine samples which he immediately sent to the lab. I had additional visits from the host and the television crew who were still astonished about how smoothly everything was going. They really wanted some drama and action!

When the eighth and final day came, I was very excited! During the last two days I actually counted the hours as I really wanted to get back to the real world and out of my solitude. Everyone came and we held a small water drinking ceremony. I was so excited that I cried in front of the cameras. It was such a pleasure! The whole experiment is documented and English subtitles have been added. It can be viewed at www.pranalife.co.il/breatharians-ray-maor-tv-project/, or at raymaor.com.

In the end, there were three sets of motivations for doing the show. My personal motivation was to open up people's understanding and rid their skepticism about how our bodies work. I also wanted them to understand how the universe works and how our consciousness and belief systems influence our bodies. The TV show's motivation was nothing more than to make an interesting, dramatic show that would bring them more viewers and revenue. The businessman was all for the science.

The only party that truly benefited from the outcome of the experiment was the show, although I still feel that we did not focus enough of the show on the deep understanding of what breatharianism actually means for our world culture. What does it mean to say food is not really necessary? What does it say about us, our spirit, our current beliefs and how this could deeply impact the world as we see it?

Retrospectively, I did not have a clue how much that show would change my life. People started recognizing me in the street asking to take my photograph and give autographs. I felt like the survivor of a reality show. It has opened up many doors for me and has given me the motivation to write this book since knowledge of this lifestyle is still missing in the world.

Other Experiments

Before my own scientific experiment, there were only two other breatharians in the world who had allowed themselves to be televised. The first and most famous one is Prahad Jani, the Indian man whom I mentioned in a previous chapter. His experiment took place in India and spanned ten days of dry fasting under medical supervision inside a hospital. It was followed and acknowledged by twenty different doctors and published mainly in the east. Westerners did not take it too seriously because it was made in India and not in the west.

The second experiment was a failed one performed by the well-known Australian breatharian, Jasmuheen. Jasmuheen is famous for the book, *Living on Light* which gave breatharian lifestyle seekers a framework and guidelines for the pranic living process. It took place on the show *60 Minutes* but the experiment failed after a few days of dry fasting. My own understanding from correspondences with Jasmuheen is that the failure was a set-up arranged by the investigative reporter and his team to give breatharians a bad reputation and to discourage the breatharian lifestyle, presenting it as fraudulent.

The show I appeared on was called *True Face*, and its host was a famous journalist in Israel called Amnon Levi. He is known to be very skeptical and a difficult man who usually finds any loophole in his researched guests' stories. I therefore, mentally prepared myself for criticism during and after the show.

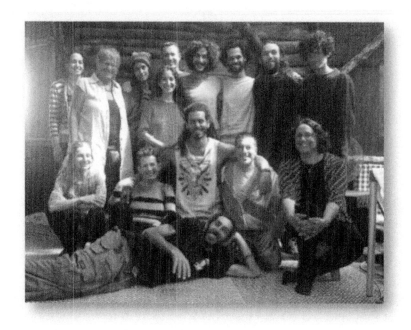

Fig. 3- The first group of amazing people to pass the Pranic Living Group Initiation

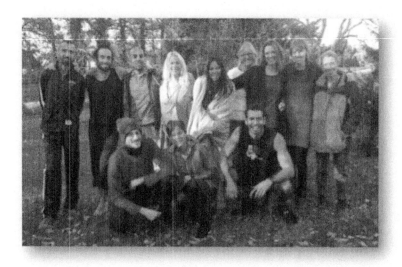

Fig. 4- Another amazing group who finished the process in Nov '15 in the Nevelands

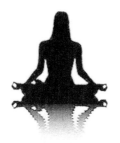

PART THREE

CHAPTER SEVEN

How To Become A Breatharian

Known Methods Of Light Nourishment

There are currently four commonly known methods for becoming a light-nourished individual. The first two methods are practiced in pranic breathing and the last two in sungazing. The methods I am most familiar with are the 10 and 21-day processes. The 21-day process is explained in *Living on Light* by Jasmuheen, already mentioned, who has told me several times that this method is no longer recommended. The success rate of remaining a breatharian after undergoing the 21-day process is approximately 10%. This is probably because the mental and physical shocks you undergo are significant and really turn your world upside down. In short, the challenges are great and only the strong-willed survive.

The third method, also discussed in a book by Jasmuheen, *The Food of the Gods*, takes several years to complete and combines a slow reduction of caloric intake, healthier eating and climbing the ladder of taste. This begins with being a vegetarian followed by being a vegan all the way up to a higher level of taking in less physical substances. This method employs many different forms of meditation and the emphasis is on *take your time, do it right*. I have personally read the book and felt that for me, the quicker method is preferable. Other methods pop up here and there. Some suggest simply reducing the amount of food we take in.

Some are quick and some are slow. The latest one I heard about is an 8-day method to reduce about 80% of your caloric intake. (I am not sure that this qualifies as living on energy).

The final method, the Pranic Living Group Initiation was developed by a colleague and I in our search to perfect the other processes, giving participants more chances of success via support. We are currently delivering it in multiple locations around the world. For further details see: raymaor.com.

Sungazing

Many books have been written on sungazing, which is better known in the world than pranic nourishment and breatharianism. I will summarize what I know in this section.

Sungazers change the way their bodies function to receive more light energy from the sun by gradually staring at the sun in a process that builds up over several years. A sungazer stares at the sun either during the hour after sunrise or during the hour before sunset, or at both times. One starts with just 10 seconds per gazing and gradually increases the time to 45 minutes per gazing. This means approximately 270 sessions reaching over 6,000 minutes of staring at the sun. It is done barefoot, staring directly at the sun. The overall process takes about a year-and-a-half depending on whether the individual has time to see both sunrise and sunset. The type of climate they are in, their spiritual level, their belief system and their unique ability to adapt, all determine their progress.

The 21-Day Process

The 21-day process was once the only breatharian initiation process and it is the one I personally underwent. Chapter 14 of *Living on Light* by Jasmuheen explains this process in detail although Jasmuheen no longer recommends it.

The 21-day process is not easy and requires a long period of mental preparation before setting the target date. There are very few people who choose to do it immediately after hearing about it. Even after you have started the process there is no guarantee that you will complete it, although statistically speaking, those who start it will usually complete it as they go into it mentally prepared and in the right state of mind.

A breatharian guide is required because it is dangerous to do this process by yourself. I know a few people who decided to ignore most of the recommendations by doing the process completely by themselves and all failed to complete it or went back to eating exactly *one day* afterwards, which I consider a sense of failure.

The Pranic Living Group Initiation I developed is much easier on the body and the mind than the aforementioned 21-day process. In the next section I describe the Pranic Living Group Initiation and I also go into smaller details about which meditations are required to be done and when. Yet I caution again,

> It is vitally important not to try to do the pranic living process alone!

The Pranic Living Initiation

I developed the *Pranic Living Group Initiation* in 2014 after gathering as much information as possible and witnessing the challenges most people face in adopting a breatharian lifestyle. The Pranic Living Group Initiation is the time it takes for the body to transform to become nourished by prana. Most initiations I teach take ten days. Much can be said about the process but I do not feel it is morally right to encourage anyone to go through the process without an experienced guide.

Most people who enter the process do not have their minds set on completely eliminating food, although they can if they truly wish to. They are more likely to be keen to enhance their spirituality, their pranic intake and their general life experience. Most who have gone through the process have cut back drastically on food and enjoyed the pranic living process togetherness. *The primary goal of the process is to enhance your pranic intake and to reach an independent pranic state.* Food reduction is one of the many valuable byproducts.

Two guides and a minimum of two helpers are present throughout the process who have themselves passed through the initiation. The major improvement here in comparison to other processes is that we focus on the success of the individual once he or she steps back into everyday life. This is because we have seen how many people face emotional difficulties or social challenges when they return to their everyday lives.

We decided to prepare them well with additional support, tools and further meetings. Another difference is the fact that the process is done in a group and not individually.

It occurred to me as a former guide of the 21-day process, that 21 days is extreme and not possible for most people no matter what their commitment levels are. In response, I made a list of all the difficulties and came up with multiple solutions. The Pranic Living Group Initiation is an answer to those challenges. The secret lies in a combination of a short dry fast accompanied with special breathing and meditation exercises which assist the physical body to completely cleanse its accumulated toxins and expands consciousness. Experience has shown that participants go through a shorter period of weight loss and physical weakness and get back to their normal strength much more quickly.

Since all breatharian processes detox the body, we ask that participants eat raw food for a week before the process and do one day of water fasting about four or five days before we start. During the process itself, participants start by eating fruit for one day, then do a three and half day dry fast and for the rest of the time drink small amounts of fresh, diluted fruit juice. There are two mandatory activities—namely morning and afternoon breathing/meditation exercises. Between these activities many optional added value lectures and workshops are offered on subjects such as learning how to manifest, achieving happiness, yoga, different art forms, Falon Gong and more.

After the process, we recommend at least two months of drinking fruit juice in small quantities. The process raises the individual to a higher frequency and causes pranic nutrition to jump up to between 60% and 70%. To complete the process, one must embrace a breatharian lifestyle for at least a few months. From what we have seen, one who passes through the first two to three months has made the consciousness leap and thereafter usually chooses to eat about 20% of their former intake. Some, like myself, decide to take it to the extreme and do an entire year of minimal physical nutrition to enhance the experience.

The process contains several long silence exercises, reminding us of the connection we have to our Higher Selves and to our future and past selves. We offer a half day 'karmic cleansing', which I uniquely developed. It involves a beautiful experience of Self-remembrance, forgiveness and gratitude that, when done in a group, amplifies the experience and connects us to self-love.

It is often said that each day in the process brings a different experience and therefore one cannot really know how it will all end. If you have had experience with other spiritual processes like dark room therapy, Vipassana,[22] vision quests or other types of long fasts, I can say that the Pranic Living Group Initiation is a combination of all of them, multiplied! It does not mean it is difficult, only that you 'jump' into a deeper understanding and your normal knowledge 'download' suddenly becomes clearer and more intuitive. During the process, the body undergoes various transformations depending on the stage you are at.

Generally, one of the greatest and most important things we need to understand when we go into the process is that the *spirit within* truly guides us. In the pranic book, *Living On Light*, Jasmuheen calls it the *DOW* (divine one within), but here I try to take a less spiritual approach and call it our 'intuition' or 'Higher Self'. This is what guides us, motivates us and sets out our path through life. It is always there, whispering words of wisdom and truth in our ears. We simply need to learn how to listen to it.

If I had to summarize the initiation process into a single sentence it would be,

I do not require physical nutrition because I do not believe so any longer.

This shift is the one with which you enter into the process.

---

[22] A retreat where the participants undergo several days of silent meditation.

Your belief in yourself and in your ability to self-persuade, to autosuggest and to be a builder of your own reality is crucial to the success of your process. The power of faith combined with this simple phrase embraces and explains a whole world of challenges and strengths.

The biggest mental challenge is to bypass habitual common sense by having a strong faith in our abilities as co-creators of our bodies and our existence. This belief is reinforced by exercises and overcoming personal challenges which we experience before and during the process. My personal game is to have my logical mind set up to deal with challenges through different tips and tricks as described in Chapter 10. But, that is just me and everyone has their own tools and understanding. Most breatharians are clearly more intuitive/right-brain oriented and do not necessarily come from a scientific world and perspective.

During the Pranic Living Group Initiation participants attend different workshops that connect them with their inner mastery. One of them is a manifestation workshop where they learn how to reprogram their subconscious mind regarding the effects of placebo and social programming and how to observe their own beliefs. Another workshop deals with understanding how to integrate the process into one's life, how to explain it to other people and what to drink in the beginning and for how long.

A very important note for readers is to understand that you cannot do the process by yourself. I know of many individuals who have tried and failed. Most of them succeeded in the required dry fast, but failed to integrate breatharianism into their lives and almost immediately went back to eating. Important knowledge needs to be transferred and the meditation and breathing exercises are vital to the success of the process.

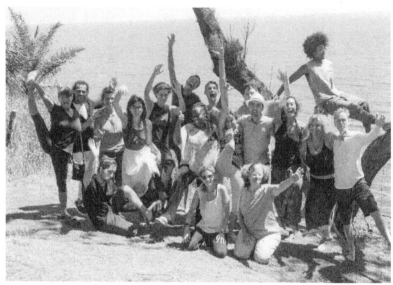

Fig. 5 - Pranic Living Group Initiation, Hawaii 2017

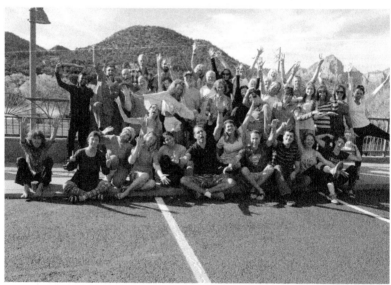

Fig. 6 - Pranic Living Group Initiation, Sedona 2017

Phases

The Pranic Living Group Initiation is generally divided into four time periods starting with the highest degree of difficulty and gradually becoming easier.

First Week

This is the air fasting week with no food or water intake. This is the most difficult period of adjustment for most; it is also the most intense period of your persistence being tested.

Days 1-3—You simply feel that you have only stopped eating and drinking. There is nothing special about these days except for your expectations of the rest of the process.

Days 4-7—The breatharian transformation takes place. These are the most special days in the process. You are required to sit or lie still for a total duration of six hours a day. You have three sets of two-hour intervals each time with an hour's break in between. During the intervals you are not to move much. You can meditate, sleep or listen to quiet music. You are to stay in the same position during each interval and try to make the intervals at the same time each day. The point of the intervals is to allow bodily changes to take place. Most breatharians report different sensations during these times.

Some have an experience similar to a kondoliny[23] (kundalini) awakening. There is plenty of time to experience these energy bursts and to deeply understand them within yourself. It is normal to go into the process with a small amount of doubt about it and yourself. This is the time to release them. In the first three days thoughts like, *Am I really ready to go through this process?* or, *Perhaps my body is not strong enough?* will go through your mind even if you do not feel hungry or thirsty.

Once the intervals begin, most likely in the middle of the third night, the sensation makes you deeply realize that a greater power than you can understand is at work. Call it what you will—guardian angels, light workers or God—something is at work that one cannot explain in a normal way. You can feel it all over your body and you learn to trust it and to let go.

I call these four days the *operation period* (as in a medical operation), since this is the time when your 'engine' is being upgraded so that you can be nourished by a higher percentage of prana. It is also the time when your four bodies—physical, emotional, spiritual and mental—are being balanced so that you are able to absorb and use pranic nourishment.

During this period you do not take any water. Scientifically speaking and according to customary beliefs, during this time you are supposed to die. However, you wake up on the fourth and fifth day and feel well. After these four days are over, you meet your guide and have a small first glass of water in a ceremony to celebrate the end of the air/water fast week.

---

[23] Kundalini bursts are bursts of energy that begin with your root chakra and rapidly climb up to your crown chakra. They rise up your spine and can last between a few hours and a few days. I have had 2 kundalini bursts in my life lasting about 3 days each time. It is unknown to me why this happens, but my intuition tells me that the frequency of the body is being elevated more quickly than the nervous system (similar to how some children's organs grow faster than they do).

You are only allowed one glass of water per hour, as your body needs to relearn how to take it in. Around breatharian circles, there is a story about a woman who did not listen to the simple rules of the process and had a liter of orange juice and died. This is a very important lesson and another reason why people should listen to their guides and to the general rules. We are playing with extremes here.

Second Week

This week is considered the *healing week* during which you recover and start drinking some fluids. The majority of people prefer water or tea but you can also drink low concentrated juices with up to 20% fruit. You are still not to move much from your location and if you have any residual energy, you need to conserve it for your body to heal from *the operation* that occurred in the first week. The healing process is already occurring and you will start feeling very different.

Third Week

This is called the *integration week* where you experience continued recovery of physical strength. You start feeling the different changes and upgrades made to your body and spirit. You start feeling better and stronger as prana has been replacing your nourishment needs, but you still need to let your body adjust to a process that can take several months. At this time you can start taking short walks according to your strength and your guide's recommendations. You can now drink a slightly higher concentration of juice. You can leave the location and even watch a 'feel good' movie once a day.

Finding A Guide

In Israel there are currently two breatharian guides of which I am one. If you are in a country outside of Israel there might be breatharians who are willing to guide you. I know there are famous breatharians who will probably charge more money (anybody hear of the term 'spiritual ego'?), but I'm sure you can find suitable people who have gone through the process to guide you.

From my understanding, this subject is best known in India and Brazil and in the west mostly in France and Germany. Of course, you can always come to Israel for a few weeks and have me be your guide.

I've wanted to be a guide from the beginning. It felt right to pass on knowledge that can change peoples' lives for the better. Hopefully, more people will decide to become guides. However, not every breatharian is suitable to be a guide and not every breatharian wants to be one. Think about it like choosing to become a priest; some people just want to have faith, while others want to teach faith.

Your guide helps and assists you through your personal challenges, guiding you through the various exercises you need to do at the right time. They show you the door, but *you* walk through it. *Your guide is in no way responsible for you!*

A person who decides to go through The Pranic Living Group Initiation is making the decision on his or her own and by the trust of their inner guidance.

You can also go through the process in Brazil for those who want a chance to get out of the country and meet a small community of breatharians. Being surrounded by a small village of people who have gone through the process themselves can be a great help for someone starting out.

Before a guide and a breatharian apprentice start out on the process they will conduct several meetings to make sure you are mentally prepared, that you are doing it for the right reasons and to ensure affinity between you and your guide. A relationship of complete trust needs to be established.

One generally meets one's guide a few times before the process and once during the process and during the first water drinking ceremony which takes place at sunset on the 7th day at the end of the air fasting week (this might change in the future if we open up a breatharian academy). Each night you and your guide will talk on the phone about your day, your emotions, difficulties and tasks. Your guide will offer advice about that day and for the day to come. We take it one day at a time. In the first week the emphasis is on talking every day. After that, it depends on both of you. From the second week on, deeply understanding that this process was up to me and my Higher Self, I asked my guide to communicate with me every second day. I found there is a great fulfillment in silence.

You have chosen to undergo a life-changing process, so this is not a good time to have ego issues. Truth and honesty about your sensations, your difficulties and your challenges is imperative. There must be *absolute trust* between you. Your guide needs to be aware of every aspect of your process to be able to give you the best advice.

To become a breatharian is to follow your inner guidance since you intuitively know many things. Going through the process gives you additional mental strength since you are embarking on something so wonderful that is considered to be in the realm of the soul and light. It is an unselfish act that raises your frequency and that of humankind. So, do not worry —you are in safe hands and are carefully watched and loved.

Finding A Caretaker

The caretaker is a person who takes care of your *physical* requirements during the process. He or she usually comes on a daily basis and stays around for a short time taking care of things like the laundry, cleaning up your environment or making juice. Even though you can do these things by yourself, the job of the caretaker also enables you, the breatharian apprentice, to constantly stay in the present moment and to preserve your energy and attention for the transformation process. Being in the moment is the key here and the caretaker assists you.

If this is the first time the caretaker is taking on this responsibility, he or she will receive a detailed briefing from the breatharian guide. This job comes with responsibility and is a role of great importance in the process. It is also an honorific role since the caretaker is part of the process and grows with you while observing the changes you go through from an objective point of view. Every person and every process is so different that it is impossible to define the exact role of the caretaker.

> *The caretaker is not the person with whom you discuss your process!*

The caretaker's job is simply to help you stay in the moment. *If you need to share, you only do that with your guide.* You can of course have small conversations with your caretaker as they are your window to the outside world.

Just remember that you are alone and that you go through the breatharian process alone. You do not need to know what goes on 'out there' (unless it is vitally important) while you go through the transformation.

The caretaker will probably ask you simple questions like if you are missing anything or if there is anything special you need. They are the ones who will bring you water (from the second week), books or missing art equipment. Don't feel bad if your caretaker does things for you that you know you can do by yourself; it is their job. Even if you are a clean freak or feel uncomfortable asking someone to do things for you, get over it! The issue at hand is not your independence; it is about staying in the moment as much as possible and allowing your body and spirit to make a large leap in your personal evolution and spiritual path.

Preparing For The Process

Similar to going traveling, one should prepare for the process and these preparations take place on every level—mentally, physically, emotionally and logistically. The preparation can take months or just a few weeks.

The preparations are required to take place consciously and knowingly and the process begins even before it 'formally' begins. On day one of the process you already need to have been there mentally. This is why, for example, I did not feel hunger or even thirst on the first day. I was already mentally ready, having known my guide and good friend and knowing what to expect.

When preparing for your process you must think about what types of issues you are going to face. You must imagine how you will deal with these issues and to consider whether they will be a problem. Your guide will be there to consult with during the process, but not to hold your hand. You are doing this by yourself.

Main Guidelines

For individual preparation in advance of the starting date there are several guidelines. Most of them are in *Living on Light* by Jasmuheen and I share some of them here:

Be prepared to spend three weeks completely outside your normal world—no phone, no Internet connectivity, no technology, no job and no social life. These are the most important requirements for you to get the full benefit of the process. Following these rules requires surrender and humbleness. Trying to cheat will only make things harder for you.

Release all thoughts and projections from the outside world; step into yourself and connect with your Higher Self.

Do not worry about anyone else in the process—your only concern is yourself. Mothers, fathers, children, family members, spouses and pets are not allowed to visit or call.

Once you've started the process you cannot worry about business meetings, payment of bills, watering the garden or pets. You need to have taken care of these things as if you have gone abroad and disconnected. It is best to find someone to take care of your personal affairs and to make sure that you have closed potential loopholes.

Surrender and hand over control to your inner guidance. For the majority, this presents a challenge. Don't forget that wherever you think your challenge may be, that is where you will be challenged!

There will be no sexual activity of any type, including self-pleasuring.

General Recommendations

Though not an exhaustive list, below are some general recommendations that you may find helpful as you journey through the process.

Music

Music is always fun and I do not know of anyone who does not enjoy some type of music. Take peaceful music to your process—classical or whatever makes you feel at ease.

If hearing house/electronic/trance music makes you feel comfortable, that also works. It is really up to you. My recommendation is that if you only normally listen to loud music, take some soft music with you as well; you might be surprised to find that you connect with it. Sounds like ocean waves, meditation music or Zen style music is great to help you stay in the moment.

Take a speaker or a good headset. If you bring a speaker or a sound system, it is better to have a remote control because at certain times in the process you should keep your body still and minimal movement is required. A remote control will come in handy at those times.

Musical Instruments

Treat this period as quality time to connect with your musical side or to start learning a new instrument.

It is recommended that you do this from the second week onwards. Bring everything you need to use the instrument (lyrics, tuners etc.). Instruments that require too much strength or breathing like a didgeridoo are not recommended at first. Consult your guide as necessary.

Painting/Drawing

Whether you have an interest and talent for painting or not, you can always keep yourself occupied and connected with paper and colors. I am not gifted in drawing, but I decided to make large geometrical shapes which turned out wonderfully. I especially focused on the Flower Of Life and other sacred geometry. Remember to take everything you need for your painting including brushes, cleaning materials and paper towels.

Juggling

If you ever wanted to learn how to juggle or do any other type of performance art, now is the time! This is not for the first week but for the following ones. There are many types of juggling to choose from—balls, pois, devil sticks and staff. You can look these up online.

Books

It is best to take as many books as possible since your moods will change and you do not know what will please you at any given moment. You can see a list of recommended reading material at the end of this book. In general, it is better not to take 'heavy' reading which will make you think too much. It is highly recommended that you take inspiring or spiritual books —the types that keep you in the moment. Your subconscious is more open to subliminal messages during these weeks.

Accessories

Include paper, writing instruments, colors, a ruler, scissors, glue, wood and anything creative you can think of. After a while creativity simply jumps out of you! Be prepared ahead of time as it will be difficult to find these things once you are there.

Other Ideas

Make balloon animals, origami, cards, play solo games or learn tricks.

Empowering Elements

If you are a new-ager consider bringing crystals or any other healing and empowering objects depending on your belief system. Bring some plants into the room or mascots and amulets that have personal connections for you.

Camera

For photography enthusiasts, you may wish to keep track of the physical changes in your body.

CHAPTER EIGHT

Mind Mastery

Understanding Mind Mastery

Mind mastery is a great topic. It is achieved when we master the observation of our thoughts and we learn to influence and understand how the mind works. With mind mastery we can achieve character changes, a high degree of optimism, gratitude and happiness and many other necessary tools to reach our maximum potential. We embrace the fact that we are creators of our own reality and we take up the reins in our lives. Mind mastery assists us in solving the different mind games in life and in particular, games that are created by the small ego. The small ego wants to keep us in our comfort zones and make us less confident of our divine intuition.

To be a mind master, one should first and foremost understand that everything we feel and think is a choice that we make with our consciousness. Most of the time we allow our thoughts and emotions to run wild and free and it seems we have no control over them.

However when we are mind masters, the wheels turn in our favor. There are different levels of mind mastery. I cannot say that I am perfect but I can say that I have reached a high level of understanding that rarely allows negative emotions to reach me. If they do, they are discharged in a matter of seconds.

Achieving mind mastery is a goal I believe everyone should strive for especially because it affects everything in our lives.

It allows us to perceive reality in a better way, to choose how we decide to envision life and to take control of our thoughts, emotions and manifestations. We need to truly practice it and make it a way of life. It starts just like any hobby and practice makes perfect. Mind mastery is not achieved by reading books.

Our brain is built like a cloud of connections between axons; each of these connections can be strong or weak. The brain works like a muscle and the best way to describe it is: *use it or lose it*. The mind is like the brain in the sense that if it does not use a particular belief system it will not generate the connections needed for change. *Our goal is to have the mind use a chosen belief system so much that it passes on to the subconscious mind.* When this happens, the chosen belief becomes completely automatic. This is what we call a *character change* or *a change in perception*. In essence, we experience a new reality. You become what it is you always planned to become.

We are talking about *positive brain washing* such as autosuggestion, affirmations, imagination and guided meditation. All these have one thing in common—they slowly convince the subconscious that something is true. This is done unbenownst to us through commercials, social rules and standards, symbols and music. With mind mastery you become an observer. You become the intersection police officer who allows particular emotions and thoughts to go into your mind while consciously avoiding others. It is a matter of observing, choosing, understanding, clarity and persistence.

To get our subconscious in on it, some writers will repeat the exact message over and over again using multiple examples and different words. A popular book and movie that uses this is, *The Secret*. You can summarize the entire book in a few short sentences but the writers and producers used a technique taken from different worlds of repetition so that the reader or viewer will subliminally comprehend the message.

The Secret is a slow, steady, positive brainwash that teaches the reader/viewer about the Law of Attraction via multiple examples and multiple speakers.

It is not my way to repeat myself and therefore I would like you, the reader, to be conscious enough to understand that if you like something you read here or any technique that speaks to you, you should assume responsibility for it. You can read it again, practice it, give yourself examples, share it with others and use any technique that best works for you to digest it and embed it into your subconscious.

This book is about assuming responsibly and understanding the power that we have as individual creators. At times this power is more than we can comprehend. I am not the type of person who will chew your food for you before you eat; I am the type who will show you your own inner strength and will believe in your ability as king or queen of your domain! We are all magnificent, multi-dimensional beings who have reincarnated here for a short period of time. I trust you to do the right thing for yourself. Assume responsibility for your life, your thoughts, your emotions, everything! Trust that you have an inner guidance that is bigger and stronger than anything external to yourself. Know that you are guided in every situation and that everything that happens, happens for a reason.

Our Comfort Zone

When dealing with spiritual growth we need to define what a comfort zone is. A *comfort zone* is the place to which we withdraw when a challenge arrives. It is where we are most comfortable and where we are least likely to grow mentally, physically, emotionally and spiritually. Our comfort zone is full of excuses; it is usually derived from our personality, education, social standards, friends and so on. For example, an individual who chooses not to keep any type of a fixed workout may be choosing to be in his or her comfort zone. It is more comfortable to be there but it is not necessarily a good place to be, especially for one's future. To constantly choose the comfort of your television set over books, magazines or other imaginative stimuli could also mean staying in your comfort zone.

Being in a comfort zone is also noticeable in small things. An example of this is when students sit in a particular chair in the first semester and then go back to the same chair in other semesters because there is comfort in sitting in the same place. We build many small comfort zones in our lives. The trick is to recognize them and know that you are not dependent on them. Good growth comes from exiting our comfort zones. Do it consciously! Recognize where yours are and go beyond their boundaries. If you get completely cranky when you are tired, it means that tiredness has bitten into you. Can a sensation or a feeling be stronger than you are?

We *choose* to feel our reactions, not the other way around. We choose and assume responsibility for every emotion we feel. When someone insults us and we get offended, is it that person's fault or *our* fault? Of course it is *our* responsibility! It is just words that have been thrown in the air and out of a person's mouth. It is easy to blame someone else for our own emotional state.

Blaming others is being in our comfort zone.
It is okay to feel negatively but we must understand that it is our own choice. We cannot blame others for what we feel. We have control over our own emotional reactions. This might take some time but when we assume responsibility for every emotion we have, we also learn that we can choose to feel positive emotions and choose to let go of negative emotions quickly and efficiently.

Learn to recognize your comfort zones and try to work on them one by one. If one of your comfort zones has to do with emotional eating, try to observe it from a third person point of view. When we become conscious that we are eating out of emotions such as loneliness, a broken heart or boredom, we tend to do so less and less. *Consciousness is the key*. Be strict but forgiving with yourself. Allow yourself to have rules but also allow yourself to bend some of them. After all, we are all evolving! Self-love is the primary goal; only after that can we truly love others unconditionally.

Your Subconscious Mind

Your subconscious is called many things. It has many characteristics and is both complicated and simple. When we say *subconscious* we actually mean the layer of the mind that we are not consciously aware of. The book, *The Power of the Subconscious* by Joseph Murphy is excellent for deeply understanding the best methods for working with your subconscious. Think of your mind as a flower and your subconscious as the ground that holds the seed. One can only see the flower but the seed and roots are where the flower's program and nutrition comes from. What we decide to seed and feed our subconscious roots is very important as it determines what we experience in our outer world.

A basic understanding of the difference between our conscious and subconscious is that the subconscious mind does not understand the way the conscious mind does. *The subconscious has no logic; it is a place of symbolism, shapes and association.* It is not a place that knows how to analyze. A simple repetition of an affirmation before we go to sleep will cause the affirmation to sink into the subconscious mind even if we do not consciously believe it. Try this for example: Take two minutes of your time now and simply repeat to yourself, *I am feeling better and better*. Say it slowly and do not change your tone (be monotonic). Let the message subliminally sink in. Give it a try right now; don't postpone! Really give it a try right now if you want to internalize this lesson.

Say it out loud and commit to the full two minutes—do not do it half way. Don't let your small ego think that you understand the lesson when you have not followed the rules.

Let's analyze what just happened here. Your conscious mind does not really believe that what you simply say will come true. These are just words tossed into the air. But what was your sensation after saying, *I am feeling better and better* for two full minutes? Didn't you feel better? This is just the tip of the iceberg. There are many NLP (neuro-linguistic programming) methods that directly touch the subconscious. Our above exercise is not one of them; it is just an example of how an affirmation, *without even placing intention* can instantly change your mood.

This example shows us a very important lesson: *what we put into our subconscious mind is what will sink in.* The words we choose and our intentions all go through to the subconscious! This is why mind mastery is so important. Imagine how many things go into our minds daily. Imagine how many commercials we see and how much violence and negativity we get exposed to and get used to. It is so much that we cannot distinguish it any longer from our normal lives. Become a mind master and see what is attempting to go through your mind; choose what you will allow through. Choose positivity and optimism instead of negative thinking. Choose to see the good things in people before you judge them on their undesirable qualities.

There is something that is called the *cocktail party effect*: Imagine you are sitting in a cocktail party and around you are many different people distributed in different groups. They are spread around sitting in different locations in the party. Each group is engaged in a discussion just like you are probably engaged in with someone. Suddenly you hear your name coming from a different group. How can that be? Your attention was fully focused on the conversation you are engaged in. However, your subconscious listens to everything continually and is much stronger than what we credit it with.

Your subconscious is like the National Security Agency (NSA), screening phone conversations for the word 'bomb'. If it hears something familiar, a red flag immediately comes up. If you hear your name or the name of someone important to you, the subconscious will listen closely. The cocktail party effect is used in marketing. For example, stores play music because they prefer that our brains not think too hard about what we buy. For them, it is better that part of the brain be used to analyze the music subconsciously so that we become a more susceptible shopper.

I have given this example to try and show how strong our subconscious is and how important it is for us to create filters for it. The main words here are *conscious choice*. Choose your music wisely as your brain will flag all the words it hears with associations, which can be negative like in rap music.[24] Choose your movies carefully as your subconscious mind will always try to identify with the different characters. Choose your friends and the people you hang out with. Learn how to use the subconscious in the best way. Learn that it is a part of you and can be used to plant new seeds if you want to change something inside yourself.

The subconscious is the ground in which we plant our seeds; it is the land that our flower eventually grows upon. Don't feed it bad nutrition!

---

[24] I love rap music melodies; there is no judgment here, but the choice of lyrics in rap music is usually not of the highest degree for our spirit.

The Power Of Words

When we are babies we do not yet think in words; our world is completely abstract. Words add a frame to our world. As we grow up we slowly change the way we think from pure thinking to inner dialogues that use words. This means we lose some of our imagination and some of our uniqueness but we gain the ability to communicate with others. When you say a word you release its energy to the outside world. The outer world is made up of the physical world we know and other more sophisticated energetic existences. This includes the existence of a hierarchy of other sentient beings like other life forms, planets and angelic like forms.

Our intentions, emotions, expectations and words are used to create our world whether we are aware of them or not. Learn how to choose your words wisely since they invoke strong symbolism in your subconscious. Regular usage of negative words such as 'hate' and 'fear' have an effect on your brain and your subconscious mind. Choose your words wisely. Train your mind to reduce the usage of negative words. Learn how to be a *yes* person who sees things optimistically.

Our words build our world and our perspectives. Using words such as *yes, abundance, pleasure* and other positive words create positive effects. Negative words bring you negative effects. When we use the language of intention, imagination and manifestation we are limited to only using words because before we learned language, our thoughts were abstract.

Language has limited our inner dialog to words. Giving compliments is a great exercise in choosing the right words. There are so many compliments we can give when we learn to appreciate the small things. And who does not like a compliment from time to time to provide our small or large ego some food?

Affirmations

There are two very important rules when choosing the correct phrasing in making affirmations. The first is that we want to state it in the *present tense*. Think of the difference between saying, "I'm *going* to have a beautiful day" and "I'm *having* a beautiful day." It is basically the difference between saying, "I *want* to have a beautiful day" and "I *know* I'm having a beautiful day." When we affirm in the present tense, we signal our subconscious that this is the one and only reality. Our life is perceived through our own two eyes; if one convinces the subconscious of what one wishes to happen in the *now*, it is received as a command as simple as that.

The second rule is: Always state your affirmations in the positive. The subconscious receives words *literally*. If, for example, you have a weight problem and you wish to give yourself positive affirmations to deal with it through intention and the use of correct words, you wouldn't say, "I do not want to be overweight," as the subject of your affirmation will be *overweight*. You would say instead, *"I am healthy, I am in shape, I am thin"*. The focus and subject of the sentence is no longer the weight.

I learned a good method from a great master of happiness. It is simple and it works! Every morning when you wake up before you get out of bed and put your feet on the floor say, "I am having a wonderful day!" and give yourself a big morning smile. Do *not* say, "I'm *going* to have a great day" or, "This day is *going to be* wonderful." The emphasis here is on the present moment and on 'knowing'. When you know, you simply know.

When you attach this affirmation to your smile (even though you have just woken up), the brain makes the connection and starts perceiving your day with a positive attitude. As we all know, a great start to the day usually brings great continuity. Try it for a few days and see how you feel with it. Understand that the power of words and positive affirmations both within yourself and in the outer world is a great instrument for mind mastery and self-improvement.

Manifestation

Understand how powerful your mind really is. In the book, *Reality Transurfing*, the Russian author Vadim Zeland explains how our mind sends out signals that are accepted by our reality on different levels.

These signals are no different from peptides or hormones signalling the cells of our body to function in a certain way. The stronger and more frequent the signal is, the stronger the 'inner cells' react to the request.

When we want to manifest we can use many different methods. Some of these methods were known and already understood a long time ago. They were used by various religions and some of them continue to be used today, however not necessarily for the betterment of the human race.

A prayer is a way of signaling the universal spirit (call it whatever fits your belief system) what we want. Using our imagination to vividly picture what we desire in specific detail is another.

The strongest aspect of these methods is *intention*. Placing our intention into the thought, the prayer and into imagination adds emphasis to what we want to manifest. The signal is 'caught' by our reality and raises the chance of it happening. This is why group meditation, group prayer and anything else done in a group creates a strong ripple in the space of variations and attracts and creates a stronger potential future in the direction the intended thought is aimed at.

Words have strong associations in your mind. When you think or hear a certain word, neurotransmitters immediately start running all over the place to close a circle and bring up a memory by association. Think about the word 'terrorist' and see what associations you get from that. Think about the word 'nature' and see how you feel about it. By knowing that everything in our mind works from word associations that connect to emotions, sensations and feelings, we can choose to unlearn and relearn the associations and cast them in a perspective we prefer to have and consciously choose to have.

If you live in a prejudicial society where minorities receive racist comments, try to see what the media or society places in your mind in association with that minority via social standards. You will probably find many generalizations. Interrogate the social standards and try to see how many of your current associations are there because of conscious decisions you have made and how many are there as a result of your education, religion or social expectations. You will find that many of your associations were not chosen by you in the first place.

This is where the process of *unlearning* begins. Unlearn as much as you can. Go back to the point in time where the associations were created and make your own decisions. If the word 'school' comes back to you as a traumatic memory, imagine a new association. This applies to everything. For the new associations to become habits, you need to repeat them and catch the previous association as it happens. Here is where mind mastery comes into play together with initial determination. Remember that you are a mind master. You can catch yourself thinking negative thoughts and replace them with good and positive thoughts in your mind.

The good news is it only requires a little consciousness and attention to get started. Once you do, you are on a roll to change your perceptions of everything. My former boss once told me, "Life is like a beehive; you need to know exactly where to look in order to see only the honey and not the bees."

Choose your perspective and change all brain connections to be perceived how you choose them to be perceived. There is so much to appreciate! There is more complexity in a single leaf than in our most complex super computers. We are surrounded by amazing human beings who share life and love with us. We have health, nature, loved ones and many other gifts. Everything we have can be perceived with wonder, amusement and joy. *It is a matter of choice.*

Practice makes perfect. We are who we think we are. Deleting old connections can be done just as easily as making new ones. When you become good enough at applying these methods, you will find that a simple intention and decision to change a thought is enough to make it happen. It is enough to tell yourself *I am happy* to create the sensation immediately all over your body and to understand that you truly are happy. When you are a breatharian, you will want to change the way you perceive food and remove old mental dependencies, replacing old connections with new ones.

The Magic Number

It is known that a new habit can be mastered by repeating it 21^{25} times. The same approximate number is used to learn a new word. One must use the word approximately 21 times for it to be embedded into the automatic brain dictionary and to use it accurately. By knowing this rule we can set up new healthy habits by focusing only on the first 21 times we do something new. Suppose that I do not really like exercising but I have decided that it is time to get back into shape. I will focus myself on exercising for the first 21 times. When I get close to that number (after about a month or a month and a half), I will notice that I am already exercising on 'auto pilot'. I will notice that I already have regular days on which I prefer to exercise and that I am not suffering or forcing myself to exercise any longer. From here on, it just becomes a habit. This can also be used to change old habits. Say I have an issue with money and that I know I am cheap. If I fight my cheapness by giving to a charity or invite my friends out and pay for others more often or do any other 'anti-cheap' action 21 times, I will embrace this new me and actually step into the new figure. It is a matter of releasing our objections born from the fear of long range commitment to change.

---

[25] Notice that the 21-day process is built in this way for the exact same reason – to break the old habits we have of eating food in a controlled environment.

We are usually afraid of long-term commitments. When a person wants to make a new habit like taking up meditation, the first resistance comes from a place of resisting commitment. You may want to do it for the long-term but getting started is simply problematic. The small ego-mind excuses and comfort zone programming starts kicking in. Thoughts such as: *I don't have the time, there are more important things that I need to do, it will take me too long to reach the high level I want to achieve* and so on will come to the surface. We humans are especially bad with commitment issues and generally like to keep our options open. When we focus instead on the initial 21 times and do not try to make a long-term commitment to something new, we feel less stressed. Divide your world in two until you reach the 21 times point and only then choose to go beyond it. Feel the change from the inside and see if you would like to continue whatever it is that you are doing.

It is preferred once you have decided to do something 21 times, that you persist. This will not only help you build a better and stronger character for yourself but will also strengthen your self-belief. We should be able to trust our own decisions and stick with them as best we can. Committing to just 21 times is not a big request and can be considered a gift from our present selves to our future selves. Reaching a goal we set for ourselves makes us feel good and provides us with a feeling of accomplishment. This raises our self-confidence and makes the next attempt easier since we already are a living example of our success. It is a great key to personal development.

Using Ego Against Itself

This is one of my favorites. We all have an ego, some bigger than others, which is fine. Everyone learns at their own pace and each lesson is learned in due time. I used to have a larger ego before my breatharian process and am happy that it has been reduced. This does not mean that I am without an ego but I'm definitely working on it.

The breatharian process allows me to see things more objectively and to care even less about others' opinions of me. I am not saying we should all achieve the highest degree of Buddhist monks—we all have a lot of work to do if we even want to come close to that. The breatharian process has given me quite a push towards humility and provided me with some of the insights in this book.

Using the weakness of having an ego to our advantage means knowing and accepting that we have one, observing it from an external point of view and counting on certain behavior patterns to persist.

Allow me to explain through an example from my own breatharian game. At a certain point just prior to beginning the process, I wanted to be a breatharian who only took in water and tea, which meant keeping to the absolute bare minimum of taste.

It sounded like the right thing to do since at that point in time I did not really understand the dependency that a normal eating person has on taste, flavor and texture.

These aspects are completely taken for granted. Even today, I still have an inner feeling that I have traded one dependency (food nourishment) for another dependency—taste. This is why I keep a steady workout of dry fasting days or water fasting days to remind myself that my main goal was to be independent of all things, just as monks who choose to separate themselves from all material possessions and dependencies on the outside world. So, say I wanted to take a taste independency challenge even though I have already put myself through many of those. I am bringing it up as an example. I would go for one week again only on water to remind myself of my independence.

The thought of challenging myself often goes through my mind just like any person who plans a potential future. Many times when we think about taking on a challenge we end up just thinking and not doing anything about it. Saying it out loud to someone you appreciate can force you to do it or give yourself that extra push. If I tell my good friend whose opinion I appreciate and whom my ego wants to continue thinking highly of me that I am planning a water fast for a week beginning this Sunday, it will strengthen my motivation.

It does not matter in the outer world if I end up doing it or not. The point is I have an ego; when I say my desire out loud and then go back on what I said, my ego will feel slightly unhappy. I will feel that I have let myself down and perhaps even disappointed myself. Going back on any of my decisions is no different from saying, "I am simply not strong enough", or providing myself with a comfort-zone excuse.

So, why not use the ego to your advantage? Why not give yourself more reasons to grow and commit yourself to a better future instead of taking the easy way out? The example I gave is just one of many ways of using the ego for the betterment of the self. Try to find some of your own. It can be admitting your mistakes and assuming responsibility even when you do not want to, or telling friends and family of your goals and milestones and setting a higher bar for yourself.

Choose To Let Go

When something bothers you there is no need to dwell on it. What happens to most people is that they keep thinking about the problem over and over again and end up digging their emotional grave even deeper. Take for example the process of solving a riddle or puzzle. Solutions are often tricky and not straightforward; you need to think outside the box. Most people start searching for a solution in the most straightforward way since it lies within their comfort zone and makes the most sense. They continue running in circles returning to the same thoughts and same possible solutions, getting them nowhere. The idea is to stop thinking completely or to start thinking outside the box.

Letting go means to understand that a solution may offer itself. Sometimes we are bothered by an issue, go to sleep and when we wake in the morning we have a solution for it. Letting go is understanding that we should make room for the Higher Self to work on a problem. Even a ten minute walk outside without too much thinking helps. Let go and place your intention on finding a solution. If it helps, be clear and say it out loud. Trust that a solution will come to you in one of many possible ways. When it does, be grateful and appreciative.

Controlling Emotions

The emotional body is one of our four bodies. Even though we cannot see it, it is real and functions as part of our individual self. A person who has a strong emotional body has control over his or her emotions. This does not mean being robotic—it means there is an additional layer of consciousness between the individual and their emotions. Emotions are a great part of the soul's experience and it is our goal as humans to maximize positive emotions and minimize negative ones. In the overall soul perspective *an experience is an experience and there is no duality/polarity; everything is accepted.*

Most of us have ups and downs and most people are not completely emotionally stable. We allow our emotions to control us instead of having ultimate control over them. For example, if a person curses you in the street even if you didn't do something to offend him or her, who is to blame? Is it really the person's fault who cursed you if you *choose* to be offended? We can always blame someone else for the way we feel but we are in truth, completely responsible for our emotional states.

Take the Dalai Lama—can you imagine him getting angry? At anyone? For any reason? You can only imagine him becoming more understanding, accepting and showing compassion for lack of love. Another example is getting pissed off on the road. Is there really anything we can do about a traffic jam? Will it matter to our emotional state if we are late when there is nothing we can do to change it?

Is there anything we can do to control another drivers' behavior? Contemplate this for a minute.

Adding consciousness to our emotional states is a key factor in balancing our emotional bodies. We need to be aware of how we feel and truly understand our emotions consciously. When we embrace our feelings from a place of understanding, the feelings are suddenly not so bad and we begin the process of healing negative emotions. If I am completely aware that I am jealous of my friend, I can investigate what I *perceive* is lacking in myself as well as the reasons for it. It helps me to learn and grow. The more we grow spiritually and understand that we are the kings and queens of our castles, the less of these situations we will have to deal with. Our karma ceases to provide us with situations we no longer need to grow from and we ascend to higher levels of experience.

Here is a simple method to teach you how to assess your emotional state or deal with it after an event. First, imagine yourself in the situation that you were in. Take a minute to feel, hear, see and use all of your senses and really step into the emotional state. Now imagine looking at yourself going through this experience from the outside. Imagine it very carefully. Describe to yourself exactly what you feel, hear and see. Remember you are the *observer* looking at the supposed 'victim'. Now do it one more time but this time as an observer looking at the observer. Imagine how this observer feels, hears and sees the situation. The farther you move away from the source the less emotionally connected and more rational you will become. Practice this in different scenarios in your life.

When we become the observer we are less uptight, we sooner admit when we are wrong and we become more rational. Recognizing when we react emotionally is the best time to self-reflect and gain control. For example, a loving couple should stop fighting after a few minutes and take a break. It is said that when our heart beats over 90 BPM in the middle of an argument we are no longer thinking rationally and should stop to calm down and rethink the situation.

These are some ways to build a strong emotional body:

1. *Assume complete responsibility* for every emotional state. This should go without saying. We are unique individuals and our life journey and manifestations are our own doing and our own responsibility. This doesn't mean you are a robot; it means assuming responsibility while allowing yourself to be present in the feeling experience.
2. *Learn and grow* from your emotional state. The second time around is easier if we completely understand the source of the emotional state the first time around.
3. *Monitor* when your ego is involved.

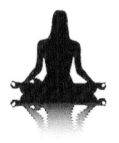

PART FOUR

CHAPTER NINE

Challenges Of Being A Breatharian

Challenges

Being a breatharian comes with a unique set of challenges. To truly understand these challenges we need to imagine what it must feel like to stop eating completely. How will our parents take it? What will we do when it is lunchtime at work? How would we go on a date? I've specified a few of the bigger challenges that I have experienced myself and witnessed other breatharians overcome.

Food

Many eating habits are taken for granted such as eating three times a day. Even a person who eats only once a day cannot easily imagine what it feels like to go for longer periods without solid food. Most people do not fast for even one day in their entire lives.

Some religions like Christianity, Judaism and Islam practice built-in fasting but many of these practices come from a place of suffering and not necessarily from a place of higher connection to God. Often a single day of fasting can result in a craving for food. Imagine going for months without your favorite food, texture, flavor or taste.

A breatharian misses food not as a source of energy but more as forbidden flavors he or she has decided to leave behind. Some cope with this challenge easily while others struggle with it. The first few months are always the hardest. During this time certain brain connections seem to break and disappear.

It is similar to becoming a vegetarian; many food sources disappear from your life and when you go to the supermarket you have a smaller selection. You see people eat meat, fish or chicken and have some recollection of what it used to taste like but you know that you have chosen not to eat these foods any longer. For a breatharian it is also like this, times a thousand!

Food is constantly all around us. People focus just about everything around food: meetings, dates, studying. This means you have constant social reminders of what you are missing. It is probably the reason why many breatharians are loners and one of the main reasons why most breatharians go back to eating after a short period of time. How would you like it if you started a new relationship in your life (prana) but your ex-girlfriend (food) is always there to remind you of your old habits? You want to move on and live your life peacefully but she keeps showing up and rubbing her existence in your face.

Obviously when you reach a balance with food in your life all of this becomes much easier, but reaching this point takes some time. One of the benefits will be that you are clear of overthinking, analyzing and comparing your behavior to others.

Social Acceptance

I would like to emphasize the issue of social acceptance when living from prana. People display different levels of acceptance and the adaptation time is individual. Most people simply aren't able to comprehend what it means because of their social programming.

I can confess that before I met my guide, even I had great doubts about the existence of breatharians as something more than just a rumor. After my television exposure it became much easier for me to be socially accepted. Ridicule turned to curiosity and sometimes even admiration.

There are generally three types of responses to the subject from a person who has never heard about breatharianism.

The first and most common response is disbelief. It is not logical after all and believing that we can survive without food goes against everything we have been taught. This is the kneejerk response from most people and they do not want to take a moment to think outside the box. The response usually comes with a type of ridicule or an expression that says, *I think you are either delusional or lying.*

The second response comes from people who understand the concept in a superficial way and can comprehend that this type of life is possible. They usually ask questions and attempt to understand what I am explaining in this book.

The third and rarest response comes from future breatharians. They want to know and experience the process themselves. They believe it the minute they hear about it and you can already see in their eyes that a change is beginning to take place.

Sometimes a person will be completely fine with the idea that a breatharian can live only on liquids and cut caloric intake to the bare minimum. However, it may be hard to comprehend that a person can survive completely on water and even without water. Each consciousness has its own limits and takes its own time to expand. If I notice that a person needs to grasp the truth step by step, I do my best to go up the ladder slowly.

The best approach for a left-brained logical person like me is to talk about numbers and scientific facts and let people do the math. If my body used up 3,000 calories a day before the process and was in balance and today receives only a few hundred calories and still remains in balance, it means that it still uses 3,000 calories a day.

The logical conclusion is that the extra energy comes from an external source. After understanding the source we call prana, I give the example of a breatharian girl in Israel who lived for a year on only water which occasionally contained mint. This usually breaks them in. When you explain breatharianism to someone, I recommend you take time to clarify all the different aspects, including the science and the spirituality.

You should expect some people to resist what you are telling them and this is completely okay. It is natural and understandable. You are bringing down a house of cards and for some people it is just too much to take in.

Social Challenges

Social challenges are considered the greatest obstacle in your life as a breatharian. In the process itself you are alone and nothing really affects you; you are with your own thoughts. The real challenge starts when you go back home and have to adjust to a new vision of yourself in your former life. A great change takes place inside when you shift to a no food mentality. It is like travelling around the world—you simply do not come back the same person who departed.

Each change that happens is for the betterment of yourself and is blessed but incorporating your new habits might be difficult where others are concerned. When you come back from the process the people around you do not know what you are going through and do not necessarily understand your quest for a higher goal. There is judgement.

One cannot simply understand breatharianism in a one-minute explanation and you do not really want to explain yourself and your lifestyle to everyone all the time. This is especially the case when you notice that most of the explanations are met with judgment, disbelief and misunderstanding. A good two to three hour lecture might cover some of the basics of breatharianism—something that cannot be achieved in a casual conversation.

Family and friends may judge you because they worry about your health. It seems not to matter to them that you feel great, have more energy than they do, your blood tests are normal and there's nothing lacking in your body. Your parents might be old-school and want to see you eat Saturday dinners with the family. Holidays can be adventurous when you tell a cousin who has not seen you for a long time what you've been up to.

This of course depends on the consciousness level and open-mindedness of your friends and family. I know an ex-breatharian who went back to eating because her parents did not accept the way she looked in the first month of her breatharian lifestyle. They forced her to see a doctor, forced her to weigh herself and she had to show her mother that she was consuming fruit drinks to make them understand that something was going into the system. This is not an easy place to be in.

For me, it wasn't a great challenge. I come from a very open-minded family. Both parents accepted my decision and we have a lot of trust in my family. I'm not saying that my mother was extremely happy to see that I'd lost almost 10 kilos in under a month but she knows I'm a grown man constantly seeking adventures and challenges. We have a mutual agreement that I can be trusted. My sister is a New Age hippy just like I am and she had heard about breatharianism before my process. We both knew in our hearts that it was possible, so why not one of us? I still think that she might one day join me in this adventure.

The social challenges usually occur at the beginning of a breatharian lifestyle when we are in the phase of limiting ourselves. For me, this first phase lasted for a year during which time I chose to exist on very small amounts of liquid and no solid food. Today, after a few years have passed, I generally eat in social situations such as the ones described above. In most social situations the simplest and truest explanation would be to simply say that you do not feel hungry.

It is our wish to be understood, to be accepted and to feel normal with friends and family. If you are a loner like the holy Indian nomads who choose this lifestyle alone on a mountain and in nature away from civilization, you do not need to worry since you will have no one to judge you. One needs to be mentally strong and know oneself to resist social standards and the need to be accepted as 'normal', to withstand ridicule and persist in one's inner knowing.

Hunger/Thirst

As mentioned previously, a breatharian does not really get hungry or thirsty. Part of the process is to understand that hunger and thirst are both controllable sensations. Where there is no dependency on food any longer there is no need to feel hungry. However, a breatharian can get hungry if they get emotional, feel bad or start eating again. The general rule of thumb is *not to drink or eat if you are hungry or thirsty* to avoid re-creating the association between caloric intake and the sensations you are feeling.

Not Feeling Full

This might be hard to understand for most people. Since a breatharian does not feel hungry, they also do not feel full. It means that if they drink or eat something they will need to recalibrate themselves about when to stop. The stomach stops signaling the brain the 'I am full' message and it takes a while to get used to this in between sensation.

Weakness

The first few months of being a breatharian might be accompanied by physical weaknesses while your body is learning how to adapt to this new energy. Each body is individual and gaining back your weight and physical strength depends on many factors such as physical health prior to the process, mental attitude and genes. A breatharian who feels weak needs to remind himself or herself that it is only temporary and will eventually pass. One usually gets back into shape between 2-12 months. I felt weak for the first 2 months but kept up regular exercise to force my body back into shape, which it did and the feeling passed. People who undergo the Pranic Living Group Initiation regain their physical strength more quickly. This is because of the breathing exercises and special meditations.

In general, our body always wants to take the easier path and the easiest path is going back to eating normally. So in the beginning, it will make anything sweet taste *really* good because it wants the immediate energy sweet things provide. Remember that this weakness is an ongoing feeling that may wear some people down and cause them to give up.

Mind Games

A mind game is a game that our ego mind plays. The ego wants to control us and there is no true spiritual growth when the ego is in control of our lives. Mind games can include anything that makes you change your mind quickly, anything that whispers in your ear, "Come on Ray, you do not really need this, give up, why are you doing this to yourself?" For me, one of the biggest mind games was the 'caloric game'. I counted every calorie going into my body, trying to understand how it was possible I was still using 3,000 calories a day while only allowing several hundred to go in while gaining my weight back! My left-oriented brain was not satisfied at all and it was starting to get to me. Other mind games can be thinking that you are not suited to being a breatharian, thinking that your girlfriend won't love you any longer and other thoughts that come from your lower self.

Learning to Let Go

A great challenge is to let go of any concerns and to allow a greater power than yourself to control your life. It is not easy for us to be humble and to admit that we do not always understand what is going on, that there may be greater and much more sophisticated things in our reality. A good example is the fact that right after the process you lose some weight. You need to be aware of this ahead of time and be mentally prepared to look in the mirror and see your skinny self which will elicit comments.

Accept that there is nothing you can do about it since *some force greater than yourself controls the process,* and that some time in the unknown future you may or may not receive some of your weight back.

Learning to completely let go and trusting a greater power is a big challenge at first. After some time, you will understand this rule can be generalized to many things in life and that in the moment you truly let go, trusting a greater power and adopting the mentality of *whatever happens, happens for the best.* Things start to change for the better. Completely let go. Trust that you are constantly being guided by your Higher Self via your intuition. Take notice when a subject comes up twice in the same day. Take notice of the people you randomly encounter in your life. What can they teach you? What can you teach them? See the lesson behind every door, even the ones you think do not exist.

Developing a Spiritual Ego

After the process you might think that your ego has been reduced as a result of some new insights, which I will not elaborate on here. A new type of ego emerges—the 'spiritual ego'. The spiritual ego is the one that tells you, "Ha, you have now attained a higher level of consciousness and understanding on how the world works, you now know how to believe in something so badly and against any logic that you are a master of your own creation and the laws of the world bend to your will and desire". So you may have just replaced your regular 'know it all' ego with another type!

This is a bit like religious people arguing about who amongst them knows the truth best. The challenge is to remain humble in front of this great power that you know nothing about and to keep reminding yourself that we are all essentially equal, we are all one. Each and every one is a soul on its journey back to the Source. I could have been the other guy just as he could easily have been me. There is no difference between any of us.

There is no right or wrong, no absolute singular truth. In addition, developing a spiritual ego might place more distance between you and others, something that existing social challenges already accomplish.

A breatharian is usually humble since he or she is required to completely let go and trust the universal spirit (inner God) for guidance on the path. Some of us develop a 'know better' attitude about spiritual development. Some really *do* know better but they probably need to be a bit more humble and quiet about it.

"Those who know do not speak and those who speak do not know."—Lao Tzu, Tao Teh Ching

Fear Of Air Fasting For A Whole Week

This only happens in the 21-day process and not in the Pranic Living Group Initiation. Even though I was a well trained faster who had been fasting for six years for one day a week on water only, I had never air fasted for more than a day. This was when celebrating Yom Kippur as a child. So this fear falls under the category of 'fear of the unknown'.

In retrospect, I can say I was not hungry or thirsty because of a leap in consciousness as well as knowing my good friend and breatharian guide who promised me that I would have a smooth ride. The only real physical effect that can annoy you is the fact that your throat is definitely dry until the seventh day and it acts as a constant reminder that you are air fasting, which causes some mind games of its own.

Boredom

Another possible challenge in some of the processes is boredom. Most people have never spent three weeks by themselves in isolation. This is not a normal state in our modern world. You don't have any communication with the outside world or any technology that connects you with the outside world. You can only talk to two people and only for short periods of time. During the first two weeks you also do not move much. One can get pretty bored under these conditions!

The process is basically a combination of Vipassana and a health fast with a long mental process of connecting to a higher power of your choice and it triples the difficulties each process inherently has. With unconditional love and a true understanding that one is born alone, dies alone and is one's own best friend, it is easy to get over the boredom.

It is wise to think ahead about what you may like to do during this time and to equip yourself accordingly. In addition, do not expect that you will sleep a lot; you will actually get only a few hours of sleep during this process. You often wake up before sunrise and will not require much sleep since you meditate often and are slowly becoming a breatharian who does not require much sleep by definition. Any and all future concerns you may bring into the process which have been created by your mind will become an obstacle and a test.

CHAPTER TEN

The Rules of Your Game

The Rules Of Your Game

To cope, a breatharian has to keep to some ground rules. For some it is easy, while others go back to eating. In Israel for example, we know of 25 people who have completed the process but only 15 are currently living a breatharian lifestyle. Try fasting for a few days through the family holidays and you'll see what I mean. If someone breaks through the first four to six months they will probably remain a breatharian.

Breatharians understand that they are playing a game inside the illusion of what we call life. A good example would be to look at physical reality in the movie, *The Matrix*. When one achieves self-mastery, one understands the great illusion better than before. You can compare this to being a player inside a computer game. This game is a part of the vibration theory in our great illusion[26] and the one who is pulling the strings is our very own all-knowing elusive Higher Self.

When a breatharian enters the game, he or she understands the human body is just one of the many existing bodies. It is the only body physically noticeable by our limited eyesight except for people who can see auras. To continue to play the game, the player must construct rules for themselves according to their understanding, consciousness level and inner strength.

---

[26] Our great illusion is an understanding that our life here is just an illusion, just like a dream and that the 'real' reality occurs between our incarnations.

Why Are Rules Required?

Think of becoming a breatharian as a challenge similar to climbing a mountain. You take it step by step and eventually get to the peak. Then you want to establish a base there and not fall down the cliff on the other side.

I have observed similarities in the ways breatharians go back to eating after the process. This can best be described by the metaphor of smoking; a cigarette smoker who has stopped will avoid cigarettes for as long as they can. Their ego will then tell them they are strong enough to smoke just one cigarette for fun, for old time's sake because of being in a social situation or because they are having a drink and the associations are strong. In that moment lies the beginning of the return to old habits and it can all go downhill from there. If you smoke a cigarette once, the next time you might tell yourself that you've already smoked one cigarette and that it wouldn't matter if you smoke another. You may tell yourself that you are completely over it and more mind games and excuses ensue.

The same goes for food. A possible breatharian narrative is that we have been addicted[27] to food nourishment most of our lives and choosing to eat something solid after a breatharian process may very well constitute 'the first cigarette'.

---

[27] Calling food an addiction is used here just to show one of the possible perspectives in understanding light nourishment. I do not use this to judge anyone in any way.

It is a good example of ego and an inability to understand that one first has to become strong enough. The recommendation is to refrain from solid food for the first six months of your breatharian life.

Rules are required, especially in the beginning.

Some people choose to continue with the rules indefinitely and then change them to suit their own experiences and personal development. Some strong individuals do not need them at all while others *think* they do not need them and find out a little too late that they actually do.

Some Examples

You now understand why some basic rules are necessary and why I applied rules to strengthen my belief system. A first basic rule will be to call drinking or anything that goes into your mouth *tasting* and not *eating*. If I were to call it *eating* or *eating food,* it would cause strong memory associations that tell my subconscious mind that I will be nourished from what I consume. This rule was created without any awareness and more or less automatically by other breatharians to avoid deep-seated associations.

When a breatharian plays their game they must always be aware of this *taste frame.* They can allow themselves to bend some of the rules sometimes and at other times apply stricter rules. I strongly believe that having rules is good for discipline and self-belief but some are meant to be broken because we are, after all, here for the experience and the pleasures of life.

Even though I have chosen a challenging journey regarding food and the world of taste as a breatharian, it does not mean that I have to be rigid. I am just one breatharian explaining his own story. Others have developed different methods of adjusting to this way of life.

Here are some basic examples of my rules in the first year after my process. I still practice some of these today, although I am less strict.

Fasting

Observe a minimum of one fasting day per week without water or any liquid. I usually do between one to two air fasting days a week. This rule is very important to maintain high discipline and is a reminder that you are living on light. In my pre-breatharian life, I used to do a water fast once a week for 24 hours to detox my body. I did this for six years and took the rule from another philosophy that recommended it. This rule is also great in case I am too liberal with myself in the days before the fast because it simply 'breaks down' everything. Once you stop tasting, your prana percentage increases and you feel your connectivity to the universe once again. This serves as a great reminder why you chose to become a breatharian in the first place.

Taste

Make taste last longer and distinguish your taste experiences from regular nutrition. You can do this by using a straw or overheating your tea or many other things that will make you enjoy whatever it is you choose to drink for a longer time. This simple rule reminds you that you are nourished in other ways than through food. You can bless the drink and take time to fully appreciate whatever is given in the moment. If you simply close your eyes you will experience a deeper flavor experience.

Tips & Tricks

1. Learn how to forget!

Some of our friends deal in the stock market. Do you ever wonder why we only remember the success stories and not the ones that fail? Try to collect memories of your own success stories in different situations, challenges and emotions and consciously forget the failures. Remember your victories and triumphs. You are not fooling yourself; quite the opposite. You are smart enough to understand how you truly function and know how to best use the brain's mechanisms to make neural connections that work for you.

2. Don't think about food

If you have decided to play this game, be completely into it and truly let go. A breatharian who feels sorry for himself or who constantly thinks, *Why can't I eat now?* or *Why have I selected this way of life?* will probably go back to eating more quickly than someone who has decided to commit to the game all the way. It is fine to question your decision as you continue with your progress but there is no reason to linger on these thoughts for long. You can always eat or drink something, just not in the huge quantities you have been used to.

3. Remember that you are *tasting*

You do not depend on whatever goes into your mouth for its nutritional value. This is an important point to remember in your game. We have a tendency to eat quickly and forget to appreciate what we swallow. Using a straw is a great way to take your time and taste something properly. Placing intention using a short sentence before you drink such as, *Thank you for what I'm about to drink* and then drinking slowly helps you remember that you have no real dependence on the drink. I know a breatharian who heats his tea to a very high temperature so he will only drink small quantities at a time. The main point here is that you are *tasting*, not eating!

It is true that a part of what we eat or drink is digested and used by the body. The amount depends on how much you choose to eat and how much your body is used to. If you choose to eat on a daily basis, your body will activate your 'food engine' and ask for more food. It also depends on where you are consciously. However, I cannot imagine someone being strong enough to eat all the time and simultaneously being able to remain in a pranic state.

4. Deal with food-related sensations

If you get hungry, do not eat; if you get thirsty, do not drink! This rule is pretty basic and ensures that the connection between thirst and hunger with food or drink will not be re-established in the brain. As mentioned earlier, a breatharian generally does not feel hunger or thirst. However, these sensations *originate in the mind* and could still occur in the beginning of the process, especially when a breatharian feels negative.

5. Learn to fake it till you make it

At least in your own eyes! Our minds do not know how to tell the difference between imagination and reality.

When you think and pretend that you are something, you actually become it for a brief moment in time. A fake smile and a real smile are interpreted in the same way and will bring up the same associations. Try it!

Autosuggestion works in exactly the same way. It is a method that relies on the belief that any idea exclusively occupying the mind turns into reality, although of course only to the extent that the idea lies within the realm of possibility. For instance, a person without hands will not be able to make them grow back. However, if someone firmly believes that his or her asthma is disappearing this may actually happen as far as the body is able to physically overcome or control the illness. On the other hand, thinking negatively about the illness (for example, *I am not feeling well*) will encourage both the mind and the body to accept and act on the thought. The main obstacle to autosuggestion is willpower. For this method to work, a person must refrain from making any independent judgment, meaning that they must not let their will impose other views over the positive ideas. Everything must be done to ensure a positive auto-suggested idea is consciously accepted, otherwise one may end up achieving the opposite effect of what is desired. We are our own worst enemies and best saviors.

6. Don't compare yourself to others

One of the biggest problems we have is the imbedded idea of *normality*. What is normal? Research done on social groups has shown that 60% of who we are is defined by the people who surround us. The fact that we want to belong and be understood makes us become more like others. This is why obesity for example, is contagious. We define ourselves according to others opinions and beliefs. The 'who's got the best grade' competition takes place from a person's birth until their maturity and teaches us to compete with others. This is simply wrong. The best thing is to compare yourself to your own highest potential and not to what others are doing.

Compare yourself to the super version of you. Comparing yourself to others causes unnecessary self-judgment and a lack of unconditional love, which is a key and important milestone in graduating to higher levels.

7. Experience food in different ways

You can experience the smell of food instead of the food itself. You can also experience food through others. Being a breatharian brings with it a true and deep understanding of the concept that 'we are one'. To understand that we are one, you must understand that the experience of one is the experience of all. If my friends are eating next to me, *I* am also eating. Sometimes I even convince my friends to eat something that I would like to have in that particular moment because I am aware that I am experiencing the taste through them.

"To be judgmental is to be disharmonious with perfection's imperfections." Source Unknown

Breaking The Rules

Being a breatharian means you have reached a certain level of self-fulfillment by consciously choosing to take up an extreme challenge. You are in high appreciation of all the universe has to offer you. Having rules is, in some way, in contradiction to the freedom your soul wishes for you. Your soul wants you to be boundless, free and full of joy. But having rules is a good thing and it is also great to sometimes break some of them.

A good example is a guy who eats raw food and becomes completely sick and tired of having organic pepper time after time. He is so locked into his world of rules that he does not even consider for a second what a good experience it would be to have a completely artificially created piece of chocolate.

It is good to have rules because they keep you in your 'frame' but you should also allow yourself to experience things as they come your way. Imagine having a task list of ten items you would like to achieve in a given day. You may strive to accomplish all of them but achieving only six or seven is also good. You may feel blessed for the ones you managed to do while being understanding and forgiving for the ones that you did not do. After all, imperfection is built into all of us and we should accept ourselves with love without self-judgment.

It is important to choose the rules you break. A breatharian should not break a rule from a place of lower consciousness.

For example, if someone is worried about how skinny you look in the first months of your breatharian life and their love and concern for you influences you to go back to eating, you might be making a choice for them and not for yourself.

Here's an example of my own rule-breaking. It happened two months after my process and I was in my office. I work in a normal job as a computer programmer and the people who work with me are also considered socially normal, which is why I decided to wait for some time before letting them know that I do not eat anything. One day someone had a birthday and was celebrating it with a beautiful chocolate cake. The group invited me to celebrate with them. They knew that I did not eat at work and concluded that I was just a health freak who only eats healthy food which I make for myself, because they had seen me drink nothing but tea or hot chocolate.

As I joined the celebration, I liked the cake that I saw. It was visually appealing both in texture and color and immediately many past memories and associations came to my mind. I knew that it was not in my rules to have cake so soon after my process. The understanding was that I had to wait at least six months before I tasted anything close to solid. I observed my mind trying to play a trick on me by rationalizing it. My ego told me I was different, special and stronger than others who had failed (remember that the focus should always be on not smoking the first cigarette after you quit!). Because I could observe my ego mind playing this game, I immediately refused. I witnessed and experienced the cake eating through the eyes and bodies of the others. Imagination is bliss!

I passed my own test with success and was happy with the results. Taste, after all, passes after a few minutes while the benefits of a breatharian lifestyle are numerous and everlasting. After the celebration I went back to my office and saw that my colleague had brought back the last piece of cake for me. I looked at it like a pirate would look at a golden treasure he just uncovered and immediately understood that I could have the cake.

The particular challenge and the right decision was already behind me.

I had already relinquished the *need* for the cake and refused my small ego. I had already observed the whole scenario from a third person's perspective.

The real thing one should fear is the habit and not the joy that the present moment can give us. Bringing the piece of cake with me to my everyday life would create a new habit, but the non-repeating coincidence of the birthday along with the fact I felt I successfully passed the test, I granted myself this surprising in-the-moment gift. The cake was wonderful and I made every bite last. I took great pleasure in remembering what semi-solid texture tastes like and the greatest thing is that it came as a complete surprise to me. After the cake, I immediately added a new rule to my arsenal: *no more birthday cakes until I am completely ready to introduce physical food pleasures into my life.* The moment was simply not the time for reintegration because I still had much to experience before getting there.

You might ask yourself why a strong person would tie himself to so many rules. What we need to remember is that in western society, food surrounds us all the time. When you simply walk down the street you are constantly reminded of food. This is not like being a recovering heroin addict who needs to meet other addicts in dark alleys in the middle of the night to be reminded of what they are missing.

The rules are logic's way of coping with the life-changing decision of becoming a breatharian. Most of them are strictly applied only in the beginning to keep yourself in the framework until you set your own 'new normal' with food, free and detached from necessity.

Discipline is part of achieving self mastery. Most of the stricter rules apply only for the first six months to one year of being a breatharian and others apply for life.

You will notice many religions or philosophies have sets of rules created for you and are often motivated by fear. In the breatharian way we are the pioneers in a largely unknown way of life, so we must develop our own rules and learn from them. Different breatharians follow different rules.

I hope you now understand why it is also important to break your rules. Not allowing yourself any flexibility will give you the bad feeling that you are being too hard on yourself and you may develop inner resistance. Having a standard set of rules is a good guideline. On my personal path, I am not afraid to change some rules or bend them to suit different situations. I am easier on myself because I rely on my inner trust and strength. Each breatharian is different but we have a universal goal: not to dive off of the high consciousness peak we have reached like the ones we passed by on our way up. As I said, I believe that, *Life is easy for those who live it hard*.

CHAPTER ELEVEN

Prana and Science

Prana & Science

To date, science has simply not accepted that breatharians actually exist. This is even after several scientific experiments were conducted, including on yours truly. There is a great German documentary on breatharianism called, *In the Beginning There was Light*. The director follows a few people who go through the 21-day process and interviews a few well-known breatharians. I am also in contact with him and we will perhaps embark on a mutual project one day.

If however, you are looking for a completely scientific explanation on how pranic nutrition works, you will not find it here. I, along with a few open-minded medical doctors, am looking for the same thing. There is no scientific explanation for many unexplained bodily phenomena. How can the body complete missing molecules by itself? Where do they come from? How can one simply drink juice without taking in any missing proteins, vitamins, carbons, etc.? How can one eat so little and still be healthy?

Presently we do not have any scientific explanations. This is probably due to the fact that science overlooks big portions of our reality—spirituality and the connectivity of human consciousness with reality. I'm sure that one day we will have more tools and a better understanding of tough-to-explain phenomena.

Just because science cannot explain something does not make it unreal.

Let's not forget that scientific enquiry keeps on overturning prior certainties, finding new explanations which show it had previously been wrong. Remember that the earth was once considered flat!

We have scientific theories but that is exactly what they are—*theories*. The Big Bang is an unproven theory as is the theory of evolution. Some of us make the mistake of listening to the theories of our high school, college or university professors as if they are the absolute truth. This prohibits objections and the exercise of our own creativity and imagination. Bottom line, scientists cannot explain everything. They do not yet know why we yawn or if our thoughts are created in our brains. They do not actually know why we sleep. Everything is a theory. Science is also based on observation and one cannot argue with an observation, which means a theory may be strengthened when there are many observations to support it. Equally, if there is even one repeatable scientific observation that contradicts a theory, the theory needs to be revised.

Prahad Jani

Prahad Jani is one of the well-known breatharians on the planet. He has followed a breatharian lifestyle for over 70 years and has reached 100% pranic nourishment. He does not require any water at all. He was tested under lab conditions, observed by two cameras and was at all times accompanied by a guard. Over ten consecutive days the observations were simple: he did not eat, drink, pass urine or produce feces. His body has reached a state of perfect recycling. The doctors gave him two daily ultrasound tests to check on his bladder and concluded that his bladder actually gained urine on some days! Amazingly, the same urine was absorbed by his body the next day through a recycling mechanism. Mr. Jani also does not sweat at all. Different sources covered the story including ABC News and I recommend that anyone who is interested in the subject search for the documentary on YouTube.

CHAPTER TWELVE

Some Thoughts And Theories

Some Thoughts And Theories

Since we cannot really measure prana, we can only hypothesize about it. We are already able to take Kirlian[28] photos of a person's aura. A Russian breatharian has volunteered to be used as an example. As expected, the results showed that her biofield,[29] which is the equivalent to a person's 'aura' was perfect and amazingly balanced.

There are not many breatharians who want to investigate this natural wonder very deeply but it is very important to me to try and understand every aspect of creation, including how matter is created out of the void. By 'matter' I mean the nutrition that our bodies require: carbohydrates, vitamins, proteins and everything else that is somehow created out of nothing when you become a breatharian. I give some theories here that my friends and I have been pondering. They are however, just theories; thoughts put into words. They are neither scientifically proven nor unproven. The purpose is to try and understand how prana fills in the missing gaps and how it gives the body what it is actually missing.

---

[28] Kirlian photography is a collection of photographic techniques used to capture the phenomenon of electrical coronal discharges.

[29] Biofield is the field of energy that surrounds each person.

Water via Humidity

I believe that when a breatharians' body is completely under water stress, it actually takes the needed water from the air surrounding the body. Almost all air has some humidity in it unless you are living in a completely desert-like climate. This could be one possible explanation why Prahad Jani can survive without water.

Perfect Recycling System

In Prahad Jani's case, the scientific study has shown that his body has stopped sweating and the most interesting discovery is that his body reuses his urine *from the inside!* This process of perfect recycling was actually observed on ultrasound! Since Mr. Jani was enlightened at the age of eight into this way of living, it might be true that his young body learned to adapt to a new way of living very early on. Younger bodies tend to learn and adapt faster.

Increase in Body Efficiency

As previously discussed, it is known from caloric restriction studies that when an animal is given less caloric intake, longevity genes like Sir2/SIRT1 are activated and the body starts to work more efficiently. From initial measurements it seems that the body initially detoxes and cleans itself; it uses up some of the collected garbage and starts to reduce nourishment more efficiently.

It is also known that the body preserves energy by not allowing all its systems to work at full capacity. For example, why should the body keep growing facial hair at the same rate if it is not a necessity for survival? In humans for example, once we start fasting our blood pressure slows down to preserve our energy levels. This is why people who fast get cold faster, get a head rush when they stand up too quickly and are generally slower.

The real question about body efficiency is, *how efficient can it really get?* Can a single calorie replace 100 times itself in a body that does not consume anything? Where are the limitations and individual borders? A normal body has a minimum level of caloric intake. Consuming more than this amount will increase fat tissues for future usage and consuming less will make the body use previously stored fat, causing us to lose some weight. Naturally this explanation is much more complex but this is its simplest form.

Filling In the Gaps

Since I personally know breatharians who have had no intake but water or herbal tea (zero calories) for over a year, I now know that prana fills the gaps between whatever the breatharian drinks and what is missing for the needs of the body. This means that a breatharian can go back to eating a very low amount of food and prana will fill in everything that they are missing in the diet. Each body takes its own time to readjust to caloric intake changes.

During my first year I measured and know that I took in approximately 500 calories per day via drinks, not including air fasting and water fasting days when I had nothing. It took my body about three months after the 21-day process to get back into shape, regain the missing weight and achieve my pranic ideal weight. Knowing this, I supposed that if I completely stopped drinking anything but water, it would probably have taken my body another three months to achieve my ideal weight and that my pranic percentage would have jumped accordingly. I would have gone through another adaptation phase. An exception to this case was when a friend of mine who weighed 44 kilos going into the 21-day process lost only four kilos during the process. I assumed this was due to the fact that she had already reached her bare minimum weight and the prana had to kick up to a higher percentage. It simply had no choice.

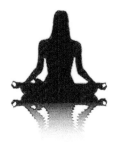

PART FIVE

CHAPTER THIRTEEN

How We Create Our Reality

How Prana, Air, Water & Information Flows

In this section, I delve a little deeper into spiritual hypotheses. My knowledge and understanding is derived from many sources—from the God within, science and from books I've read. My search for knowledge and a deeper understanding of how things really work in the world started about 14 years ago. I estimate that I've read over 200 books on these subjects—some scientific and some philosophical. I can't say I know everything but I can share some of my conclusions. I recommend you read these books—see Appendix A.

This section was written for the reader to understand how each of us can influence the world around us and realize that the spiritual world and the scientific world are two aspects of the same reality. I cannot describe all the information I have since that would deviate from the subject of the book, but I can generally describe what I understand.

Vibration Theory and Our Great Illusion

If I were to tell you that you are a prisoner, would you believe me? If I were to tell you that the matrix is real and that we are trapped by the illusions of our physical senses, would that make sense to you?

Our eyes are built to see a certain spectrum we call 'visible light'. Our ears can only hear certain frequencies in the electromagnetic spectrum. The same goes for our other senses and we perceive our entire world through them.

Did you know that a person sees about 25-30 frames per second? When we create a movie, we make sure that each second has 30 frames. If a fly, for example, were to see one of our movies, it would see it frame by frame similar to us watching a movie in slow motion. This is because a fly has the ability to process many more frames per second than a human.

So, what happens between the frames? What is the commotion about 11 real dimensions in mathematics? What is the talk about oneness in quantum mechanics? If we take a single second and split it into a million equal pieces, where are we in between these 'reality frames'? There are many questions that we cannot even begin to understand the answers to.

Even when our scientists try to dig deeper they risk becoming outcasts from the scientific community; their budgets are reduced and they could lose their mainstream positions.

Research subjects such as UFOs and unexplained mysteries are ridiculed in the scientific community even when the mathematical probability of us being alone in the infinity of space is slim to none.

The vibration theory explains that we are inside a 3D world contained inside other higher frequencies organized in a consciousness field that is layered like an onion. Each consciousness field contains and is above the lower frequencies, yet below the higher frequencies. We belong to all lower and higher frequencies simultaneously, but our current 3D body and mind are tuned to a single television station frequency inside the layers of the great onion.

In the astral planes we connect with parts of ourselves that are already in the higher frequencies which allow us to sense how different parts of us exist outside of time and space. Each frequency band (range) has its own uniqueness and rules. Our rules belong to a 3D world.

This basically means that we are playing a repetitive karmic, or cause and effect game. Reincarnations and experiences are our returning path back to the Source.

Our higher purpose is *expression and creativity*. We perceive things here in duality: right/wrong, positive/negative, male/female, giving/ taking and so on.

We have free will embedded into our system to allow for maximum experience, flexibility and other unknown factors that enter into our reality. We see our separated self as the one reality, while in truth we are each a single conscious cell working in a greater conscious body. We perceive time as moving at a linear slow speed and are fooled by our senses.

In higher frequencies, time is experienced as a single infinite moment. This is the reason why we always search for a beginning and an end. This is the last frequency of complete separation from one another. Our world and our reality is considered a place of learning. These are the general highlights of our rules. The good news is from here we can only go up.

You can imagine this world as a computer game and yourself as a player in it. Your soul is one of many who are holding the remote control for your player, your physical body. You have free will. This rule is mandatory for gaining individual experience and thus for the collective whole.

You can make certain selections as you play but there are fewer options that your Higher Self will create, since it has one main path for you to follow—the path of your soul.

The selections you feel inside your 3D reality—the ones that come from your intuition—are the choices through which you are guided by your Higher Self. We are all on a long journey up the frequency ladder back to the Source. To get there we must go through all the games which we have placed here ourselves. We are not alone. There are others helping and guiding us.

We are also not what we see in the mirror—we are *much* more than that! What we see in the mirror and what we call 'I' is just a glimpse of our true, ominous, magnificent, multi-dimensional selves.

Don't let the physical reality illusion trick you. Connect with your inner senses and keep reminding yourself that what you perceive through your senses is just a portion of the whole story—and a small one at best.

Everyone is on their way up the consciousness[30] mountain and each person has their own path and travels at their own speed. Every day brings new lessons and every day when we wake up we are slightly different from how we were the day before. Even on days when we do absolutely nothing, we learn something new. The same goes for our soul. Each reincarnation teaches us specific, pre-planned milestones to be attained. After each reincarnation we absorb our lessons—good and bad—and set off on another journey, another *re-set*. We do this consciously and out of choice and with an understanding of how the godly hierarchy exists in service to a higher purpose. Eventually, when we are done with the harder lessons we start reincarnating into lives that are full of love, self-fulfillment and happiness. Slowly yet steadily, we work our way back to the Source. The 3D reality is soon[31] to be completed on our planet and we will graduate and move up the ladder to a higher frequency. This new frequency also has its own rules, some of them similar to what we already know and some different.

Manifestation, for example, is something we control consciously and unconsciously—directly and indirectly. When I say *manifestation*, I mean our unique ability to create our own world as we see fit, given the changing factors of time.

---

[30] Read the book, *Children of the Law of One And The Lost Teachings Of Atlantis* by Jon Peniel. It contains a beautiful description about the mountain of consciousness. We all started in unity at the peak of the mountain. We have all chosen to jump off it to experience what it will be like to rediscover it. We have chosen to build our game/illusion, wipe our memories and relearn it time and time again.

[31] Soon = relative. A minute can be a lifetime for a virus, while a year can be perceived as a second for larger, different type of conscious entities like the Sun or Gaia.

Like in the well-known documentary, *The Secret* which speaks about the Law of Attraction, the physical world and human consciousness are intertwined. Try to imagine that and deeply understand what this means. Can you imagine if there were no sentient beings to observe the world, the world might not exist at all? Have you considered that if a tree falls where no one witnesses it perhaps it did not really fall?

Before we continue, let's go back a moment to our computer game allegory. As a computer programmer, this is easier for me to explain and understand. In a normal computer game the player is inside a world created by the programmer (let us not go into who the programmer is right now). Imagine a player is going into a hallway. He is walking down the hallway and sees a door on his left and a door on his right. He turns left to face the door. Now the real question is: *If the player faces and views the door on the left, does the door on the right still exist?* It still exists in our minds since we have just seen the door on the right but the computer itself has removed it from memory (existence) as it is not displayed in the current moment for the player to view. It will only be displayed if the player chooses to turn right again and see it. Do you get it?

This subject brings many complicated questions into our reality since it has been proven that reality is altered and changed by an observer[32] in scientific experiments. In quantum physics one can only know either the velocity or the position of the particle and this information is attained by measurement (meaning observing). Let's raise some unanswered questions and ponder some options.

If we are indeed living in a unique and predesigned consciousness karmic game that we've all agreed to, contribute to and play in and we have chosen to forget our true goodness for a small period of our endless lives, what happens when a person (aka the player) closes his eyes for a second?

---

[32] See *Schrödinger's Cat* paradox.

Does the world around him continue to exist if he is not watching/observing it? Where is the world around us in between the frames we perceive? Where do electrons spend most of their time? What is time? Who are the other players? Do the stars and the sun really exist or are they a live feed from the illusion? Are all scientific measurements just our expectations of what they should be? Do they help us to better understand the illusion that we initially created to experience creativity through free will?

Understanding manifestation and the creation of reality will assist some breatharians on the path. Some do not know exactly how it works scientifically but they know intuitively. The words we use, the thoughts we think and the emotions we feel all have a very strong impact on our lives and our reality. Choose your words as carefully as you choose your friends, your music and even the movies you watch. They all have a deep impact on your life and consciousness.

When we try to see our lives as part of a great illusion guided by our Higher Selves, we stop fearing death and start to understand the illusion itself. We start going inside ourselves to seek our multidimensional Higher Self. Our Higher[33] Self guides us—It knows more than we do and has planned our paths for us. There is a higher truth which is hidden from our separated ego self. Our Higher Self is in a place of unity and all-knowing where there is no separation.

There is no division, no time and no duality but here in our 3D reality, duality rules. Men and women represent this duality through logic and emotions, separation, positive and negative. In the Higher Self there is only oneness. There is no past or future—only a single, everlasting present moment.

---

[33] Our intuition is known by many names. Higher Self, divine intuition, the God within, the subconscious, the field of unity, God, the light workers, guardian angels and many others. It is important to understand that we are talking about the same thing.

Our Higher Self experiences all our lifetimes on planet Earth in the exact same moment. This means that a reincarnation in Ancient Egypt happened in the exact same time as a reincarnation in the Second World War. There is no beginning and there is no end; it never existed and it is a part of the illusion. Understanding this requires thinking outside the box of our reality. It requires thinking about time as a property of existence and not as a constant as we treat it within the illusion of reality. It cannot really be understood on a mental level.

On our way up the frequency ladder we have certain milestones, certain points in time when we understand things and change accordingly. Having problems and issues and solving them adds points to our game of soul growth. Being static in our game is simply boring and we can go through a lifetime without doing anything and ultimately make little or no soul progress. The real wonder happens when we *wake up*, similar to experiencing a lucid[34] dream. In a lucid dream the dreamer wakes up while in the dream and realizes he or she is dreaming. We suddenly realize that we are actually playing a game and that nothing really matters in the grand illusion. The player also discovers that in the rules of the game he or she is an active player and builder of the game's reality. He/she then further learns how the game of reality works. One of the rules of the game is the karmic rule; whatever you give or take comes back to you in one way or another. How you think or perceive your life is what comes back to you. Positive and negative actions and thoughts are manifested accordingly.

---

[34] A lucid dream is a dream in which the dreamer is conscious that he or she is dreaming.

Manifesting Guidelines

At this point I would like to say a few words on the great subject of manifestation. It is known that we humans manifest, or create our existence. The New Age word *abundance* and the phrase, *I am manifesting* did not arrive by chance. They are words used to create individual reality. A person who thinks about and is afraid of being sick will invariably get sick. A person who lives in the lower frequency of fear will eventually manifest what it is he or she is afraid of. Our thoughts are waves of potential. The waves can be strong or weak—there can be many small waves or large ones. In the past, manifestation used to take weeks but today, with the changing winds of our frequency and the great changes that started to occur at the end of 2012,[35] manifestation occurs much faster—sometimes in a matter of minutes, hours or days! It does not matter if you believe this or not; these are the rules of the game. You can only choose to be a conscious player and learn to control your manifestations.

A manifestation can be stronger when:

1.   *A strong emotion is attached to it.*
2.   *It is a part of a group manifestation.* In this case the manifestation power is synergetic, meaning it is more powerful as a group than in the sum of the original individuals. This is how a small group of people can influence and cause great changes.

---

[35] The end of the year 2012 was symbolized by the Maya as the end of a great energetic era and a beginning of the human Golden Age. One can compare it to a seasonal change where the human race is becoming more and more conscious of itself, more connected to Earth and is in better harmony with itself and Nature.

3. An *unselfish* manifestation is stronger than a selfish one because it carries the high frequency of love.

4. *The stronger your faith in your ability to manifest and change reality, the stronger your manifestation will become.* You will learn more about faith in the next section.

5. *Your belief in your inner strength and in your divine Higher Self* plays an important part. There is a greater power at play here that is bigger than any of us. You need to trust it. You must also start to know that there is a lesson in every scenario. There is a reason for everything and everyone you encounter in your life. The reasons might be impossible to understand in the moment and you may not always understand why things happen the way they do.

6. *Repetition, affirmation, intentions, prayers and belief* all play a role in your manifestation. If you just say it once it will be like throwing a small pebble into a large lake. If you continuously throw small pebbles you will eventually create a wave of change. Your belief in your powers as a creator of your reality will increase more and more and you will find that you are jumping levels in your game faster than before.

In the next band of higher frequencies, manifestation occurs immediately. This creates concerns around having free will. If an individual is not conscious enough to control their negative thoughts, they might cause a disaster. Imagine a helicopter controlled by the pilot's thoughts with no manual controls. The pilot must be thoroughly trained to not think negatively. What if the pilot suddenly thinks, *Oh damn, we are all going to crash!* This is why we are going through a consciousness shift in our 3D reality right now. Some people are born with a higher understanding of how things work outside our little bubble. To enter the next spectrum of frequencies we must be pure in our intentions, have higher knowing and higher consciousness. We can't enter with fear since manifestation is immediate.

Science cannot measure our 3D world because it cannot measure a frequency with tools which only work in the same frequency. We cannot see our reality from the outside. This highlights many issues in our reality and many unexplained phenomena that concern the human mind like telepathic abilities, telekinesis and other phenomena which have been removed from the public eye and moved deep underground to be used as military or private resources. What was discussed in this chapter is just the tip of the iceberg. We require much more information to fully understand our unique selves and the world we are part of. I have brought up the subject to assist in understanding how reality is manifested and why breatharianism works. For those with an open mind and a quest for truth, I recommend the reading list in Appendix A.

More Key Factors in Manifestation

• *Our physical reality is merely a reflection of our strongest beliefs.* The source of our beliefs is not always conscious, meaning they could have come from social standards, habits or family.

• *Make sure you ask for the end result and do not dictate the path* to your manifested request. All the details will organize themselves accordingly with the least resistance and according to other people's manifestations. This means there will be synergy and your manifestation will align with other people's manifestations in harmony.

• *Reality does not support you; you support reality!* If you support your reality, reality will reflect what you give it. The power of manifestation is derived from within and not from the outside.

• *Any reality is possible.*

• *The more you support your reality the more it will manifest.* The more you doubt it the more the chances of it manifesting will decrease.

• *You do not exist **in** physical reality – you **are** physical reality.*

CHAPTER FOURTEEN

Conclusions

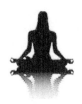

The 4th Edition

This chapter has been added in the 4th edition of this book and I am writing it many years after the 1st edition was written in 2013. In this chapter I will cover what has happened to me and what I have learned about people who do the Pranic Living Group Initiation. It can help you decide if this is your path as well.

Over the last few years I have had many breatharian deciphers. Ever since we created the Pranic Living Group Initiation (see Chapter 7), the demand for this unique lifestyle has increased. The world has changed right in front of my eyes and it is a beautiful sight!

When I first created the Pranic Living Group Initiation, I had two Q&A conversations with the entity *Bashar*. I still had many questions and wanted to get the process as perfect as I could. During our conversations I asked Bashar if the pranic living lifestyle is the future of humanity. He said in 50 years 10% of the population will be breatharians living mostly on energy. This is not far from the amount of vegans and vegetarians right now.

Fifty years ago if someone told you that they didn't eat meat, it would have been considered weird. Today, if someone told you they eat only once a week, it is considered impossible.

Since the time of the first revision of this book, I have changed much. I got married and now have a baby girl who is only a few months old.

The shift in my awareness has been mostly emotional. I noticed that my spiritual, mental and physical bodies are very strong and even powerful, yet my emotional body was lacking. So, I started doing more of the work that needed to be done on my emotional body and with the help of my amazing wife, I now feel much more complete.

The Pranic Living Group Initiation I teach has been upgraded as well. Now a team of professional healers work with me wherever I go. The larger the group the easier it gets for the participants to go through the process. This has to do with the group energy and with their intention.

I have witnessed many healing miracles occur and have taken participant surveys to make sure that we are always up to speed on demands and expectations.

I have kept my regular job as it reminds me of the reason why I am here—to bridge the spiritual and the material, the west and the east. I show that a normal person who has a normal job and a normal family can indeed take an out-of-the-ordinary spiritual path in life and set an example for others. It also allows me to bring more awakening and consciousness into peoples' lives.

Since I travel once-a-month for a week and a half about eight months a year, I really don't know why I haven't been fired yet. I work about three days a week and I am really enjoying myself! I think if we all worked a little less we would remember why we chose our job in the first place.

What I did need to do is work on my humility. I now understand why in Buddhist traditions, every student has a master. The master reflects to the student where his ego introduces itself instead of his true Higher Self. Since the release of this book and my television debut, I had more prime time television exposure where I participated in a six-week reality show called *Amazonas* to demonstrate we breatharians exist. It was a great success! I was on a roll and forgetting my spiritual self, I concentrated on a relationship with one of the participants in the show and on being a celebrity.

The time of me being more materialistic was limited to just a few months and wasn't very enjoyable. I soon bounced back to my true self. I have learned much about myself and especially about the separation of what my ego desires and what my heart truly desires. All is perfect and it is a lesson that I am still learning to this day.

My ability to bring in new information has also increased significantly and I can say I am almost channeling it through. My guides keep telling me that the best way for me to communicate with them is when I am in a state of serving others. With every workshop I teach, I feel much more in tune with my divine spirit.

The ability to bring in new information doesn't make me a genius—it just gives me many more answers to the questions I keep asking myself. In addition, I have almost completely stopped reading books.

Time, and the experience of time has altered for me. I no longer know or care what day or hour it is. Everything seems to be in a constant flow of positive change. If I catch myself thinking about the future, I take a long pranic breath and come back to my center. Not that it is wrong, it is simply not a good use of anyone's time to be in an illusion of something that hasn't happened yet. Time is a tricky thing but it is a major part of the matrix-style illusion we have been building for ourselves.

My intuitive feeling about the future is that I am being trained to be a representative of something bigger. I have always asked myself where my wonder about life in the universe came from. At the age of fourteen I started reading the *Law of One*[36] material and was attracted to it for some reason.

---

[36] The *Law of One* books were channeled by L/L Research (Carla Rueckert, Don Elkins, and Jim McCarty) between 1981 and 1984. The books (there are five) can be purchased from L/L Research's online store or freely downloaded from their library.

My favorite show was the X-Files. I am sure that you, my reader, have also gazed into the sky and felt a strong family connection with something that cannot be explained. Perhaps some truth that we decided to forget for a given amount of time until we are mature enough to internalize it in this body and in this reality?

My intuition tells me that there is something big coming in the next decade or so—perhaps a first official encounter with ETs or inner earth beings. I intuit that I will be needed and a contract that has already been signed by my Higher Self will be fulfilled. What position? I have no idea—I can only imagine! It makes me happy though when I get that intuitive message.

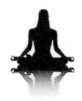

Thinking This Is For You?

If you think that living on prana is for you then you are reading the right book! I want to share with you below some of the difficulties and what most seekers want to know before they choose their next step.

Don't even think about doing this alone!

The first thing is the small ego. You know the voice that tells us that we can do everything alone just because we saw some video on YouTube? Many light workers try to do the pranic transition by themselves and fail. It is best to wait to do the Pranic Living Group Initiation in a group. There are multiple breathing techniques, workshops and guided meditations you will need to know. In addition, the group intention and energy that is required will assist the process tremendously.

This cannot be taught in emails or in videos. This is why, when I have been asked to create a video series on the Pranic Living Group Initiation, I have refused because I know it simply doesn't work.

A bad situation occurred in Australia when a woman died doing this alone and it was blamed on Jasmuheen's books and guidance. I do not wish to ever be in that situation and therefore, careful guidance and foresight is imperative.

I also wanted to do the process alone and was encouraged by my small ego, but I was convinced by my own guide and mentor that it is simply the wrong way of doing it.

The desire came from my small ego and it was to save a few dollars. It completely neglected common sense. The breatharian process is meant to be a transfer of knowledge and energy on multiple levels including the energy of the guide that is meant to transfer it. Don't overlook this. You will regret it.

Learn from those that came before you

When someone asks me to guide him or her remotely, I understand they think this is just knowledge that is being passed on. That is a very 3D way of thinking about it. Every day in the Pranic Living Group Initiation there are six to nine hours of workshops, guided meditations, breathing techniques, physical exercises and more. This cannot be taught remotely nor should it be!

Join a proper initiation! I know it is sometimes less affordable and I understand. Think about this as a once-in-a-lifetime investment in yourself.

Choose a guide that you connect to

Currently there are not many guides in the world that do this. That might change. The most important thing you should do is listen to your heart. See some of the guide's videos, read some of their texts. See if they fit energetically. It is not easy to locate guides. Best is to try and contact other breatharians from your country online. I hold several retreats every year in different countries and try to put as much information online as I can via my YouTube channel.

There are two types of guides. Those that work from the gate of the mind and those that work from the gate of the heart. They hardly mix. This doesn't mean a mental guide will be heartless or a heart oriented guide will be without sense. It means their dominance will be different. If you are looking for explanations and you need logic to fulfill your transformation, then chose a mental guide.

If you feel that you are only heart oriented and will trust your feeling to satisfy your needs, choose a heart oriented guide. As you can probably guess, I am a mental guide. I seek information, logic and experiments in my own growth and that is how I teach. I require a balance between the heart and the mind, between logic and intuition. Both need to be present. I am very spiritual but I will not use only spiritual explanations or use abstract wording like 'energy'.

What I heard from many breatharians that tried different programs is that they were missing two important things: more explanations and information about integration. That is why they ended up with me and my team.

Integration

As you have probably understood from the chapter about the difficulties of this path, you need to be ready for the integration.

Check out some of my integration videos online. They explain much about the difficulties most people have.

My friends, the initiation is really the easy part! If you are properly prepared the integration won't be that difficult. However, don't be fooled to think you can do it just because many others do. You will have mind games and social issues just like the rest of them. Your home might not be prepared for this transition, your spouse or mother might resist and many issues will come up. Most of them we can predict and we will discuss in the workshop.

Your first step is not jumping to 100% energetic nourishment. It is the initiation that switches the physical nourishment, making the energetic engine the primary one. You may still need to drink juices but reducing it by 60%-80%, which is a lot!

When the switch happens your body will no longer signal that it is hungry. From then on it is important to know that if you are a westerner, you have stress in your life—stress from relationships, work and obligations.

If you would have had the chance to live a year in the Himalayan Mountains and meditate, striving for the ultimate could have been possible. As you are not in the Himalayas and if you have one leg in a western normal life and the other leg is seeking truth and spirituality, I highly recommend not to try to make the bigger jump to strictly prana just yet. Wait a few months, integrate the first step properly and then see what your heart desires.

The initiation will change you!

We had a 91% *yes* response to our survey question, *Has this process changed your life?* Even if you think you know yourself and you probably do, don't make any decisions until the end of the process.

How to prepare for the transition

There is no need to prepare yourself much. Let the workshop do what it is meant to do. The only requirement I ask of you is to do a raw food week before the workshop to assist you with the detox that will take place. That is it! No need for pranic breathing, no need for two months juice fast or anything like that. Quite the opposite. It is a good time to enjoy the solid food you like because after the workshop you will take time off of it. It is a good time to say goodbye to some nasty habits you have picked up. Most people will give up meat, smoking and self pity after the workshop. It simply happens by itself. You can't expect to heal yourself of the deepest addictions without allowing other, lighter issues you have picked up.

Go for it!

If you feel an inner calling that is absolutely clear, go for it! This is what is going to happen when you finish reading this book—you will either tell yourself, *Ha! It's nice that this exists, but this journey is not for me,* or you will be all excited and say, *I'm going to master this amazing technique!*

Either way, if your higher guidance wants you to go you will be reminded of this randomly throughout your days. It can come in a dream, another conversation or in an online video. You will suddenly meet or hear about people who have transitioned to this lifestyle. You will find that you are thinking about it arbitrarily throughout your day and will have no idea how the idea came to your mind. This is how it starts. You can ignore it or you can see it as an intuitive sign.

Commit to your divine contract to experience this and take the first step to organize your life to go in that direction. You will feel an immediate shift with your relationship with food. You will feel less hungry and more energy will start to flow. This is the beginning as a preparation for your transition. You will then recognize the inner call for awakening through this journey.

It is not about the food!

It is not about the food, my friends. The food is only a method of understanding our desires, our stories, our 3D reality, our beliefs and our body. The food is the tool we use to get to the higher frequency and become more aware of who we are, the state of our being and our thought process.

Whoever you are, I love you as a brother and sister of light. I am happy we have come here together to experience this amazing shift and ascension and perhaps one day in this incarnation, I will have the pleasure of meeting you face to face.

With love and light,

Ray

DISCOVER THE UNIMAGINABLE WORLD
OF PROVEN ENERGETIC NOURISHMENT

RAY MAOR

Acknowledgements

Writing this book is harder than I thought and more rewarding than I could have ever imagined. None of this would have been possible without my best friend and the love of my life, Ania.

She has stood by me through difficult and challenging times and continues to support my teachings even when it takes a personal toll.

I'm eternally grateful to my teacher, Tal Gilboa who has introduced me to this lifestyle and has tottered me through my initiation.

A very special thanks to the four different editors that have helped improve my English skills and made the book readable and enjoyable.

A great appreciation to the country of Italy where I travelled while writing most of the content of this book. To the challenges of being a young breatharian while being tempted by your amazing pizza's and ice-creams.

Ray Maor

Contact Information

Email: maorray@gmail.com
Web: https://raymaor.com/
Skype: maorray
Youtube: https://youtube.com/maorray
Pinterest: https://www.pinterest.com/raymanoflight/
Facebook: https://facebook.com/raymaoreng

Appendix A

Recommended Books

Prana/Breatharian

Living On Light — Jasmuheen
Food Of The Gods — Jasmuheen
Lifestyle Without Food — Joachim Werdin
Initiation — Elizabeth Haich

Other Inspiring/Spiritual Books

The Power Of The Subconscious — Joseph Murphy
Children Of The Law Of One—Children Of The Law Of One
The Seven Laws — Deepak Chopra

Channeling Books

The Law Of One (Spirit Names Rock)
Message From The Pleiadians — Barbara Marciniak
Seth Speaks — Jane Roberts
The New Lemuria (Series) — Aurelia Louise Jones

Appendix B

Additional Resources

Prana

Product Nourishment—Nutrition For The New Millennium, Jasmuheen, Ch 4
Chariot, Drunvalo Melchizidek's Teachings, Bob Frissell, Episode 12
www.10 dayprocess.com — My English Website
www.pranalife.co.il — My Hebrew Website
Yoga Magazine—http://www.yogamag.net/archives/2009/haug09/prana.shtml
Vedas, The Sacred Texts Of Hinduism—http://veda.harekrsna.cz/encyclopedia/prana.htm

Breatharian

Breatharian Institute of America—http://www.breatharian.com/wileybrooks.html
Jasmuheen's Breatharian website—http://www.jasmuheen.com/living-on-light/breatharian*—has many video interviews with different Breatharians

Nutrition Advice From the China Study, Tara Parker-Pope, The New York Times, Jan 7, 2011
Wikipedia page about The China Study—https://en.wikipedia.org/wiki/The_China_Study

A Year Without Food

Printed in Great Britain
by Amazon

64298663R00122